Revisioning Women and Drug Use

Also by Elizabeth Ettorre:

MAKING LESBIANS VISIBLE IN THE SUBSTANCE USE FIELD

REPRODUCTIVE GENETICS, GENDER AND THE BODY

BEFORE BIRTH: Understanding Prenatal Screening

WOMEN AND ALCOHOL: From a Private Pleasure to a Public Problem?

SOCIETY, THE BODY AND WELL-BEING (*with K. Suolinna and E. Lahelma*)

GENDERED MOODS: Psychotropics and Society (*with Elianne Riska*)

WOMEN AND SUBSTANCE USE

DRUG SERVICES IN ENGLAND AND THE IMPACT OF THE CENTRAL FUNDING INITIATIVE (*with S. MacGregor, R. Coomber and A. Crosier*)

LESBIANS, WOMEN AND SOCIETY

Revisioning Women and Drug Use

Gender, Power and the Body

Elizabeth Ettorre
University of Liverpool

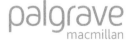

First published 2007 by
PALGRAVE MACMILLAN
Houndmills, Basingstoke, Hampshire RG21 6XS and
175 Fifth Avenue, New York, N.Y. 10010
Companies and representatives throughout the world

PALGRAVE MACMILLAN is the global academic imprint of the Palgrave Macmillan division of St. Martin's Press, LLC and of Palgrave Macmillan Ltd. Macmillan® is a registered trademark in the United States, United Kingdom and other countries. Palgrave is a registered trademark in the European Union and other countries.

ISBN-13: 978–1–4039–2174–1 hardback
ISBN-10: 1–4039–2174–1 hardbə.k

This book is printed on paper suitable for recycling and made from fully managed and sustained forest sources. Logging, pulping and manufacturing processes are expected to conform to the environmental regulations of the country of origin.

A catalogue record for this book is available from the British Library.

Library of Congress Cataloging-in-Publication Data
Ettorre, Elizabeth, 1948–
    Revisioning women and drug use:gender, power and the
    body/Elizabeth Ettorre.
        p.   cm.
    Includes bibliographical references and index.
    ISBN-13: 978–1–4039–2174–1 (cloth)
    ISBN-10: 1–4039–2174–1 (cloth)
    1. Women—Drug use. 2. Drug abuse. 3. Feminism. I. Title.
    HV5824.W6E88 2007
    362.29'12082—dc22   2006052773

10   9   8   7   6   5   4   3   2   1
16   15   14   13   12   11   10   09   08   07

Printed and bound in Great Britain by
Antony Rowe Ltd, Chippenham and Eastbourne

In gratitude to my dear mother, Helen Ettorre, who taught me a lot of things about life, especially the importance of being a good enough woman.

Contents

Acknowledgements

In the process of writing this book I have benefited tremendously from intense sociological discussions with many colleagues: first and foremost Irmeli Laitinen at Share Psychotherapy, Carol Sutton, Tracey Collett, Malcolm Williams – all from the University of Plymouth – Barbara Katz Rothman at Baruch College CUNY Graduate Centre, Susanne MacGregor at the University of London, Geoffrey Hurt at the Institute for Scientific Analysis, and Deborah Steinberg at the University of Warwick. I would also like to thank the many women drug users who have discussed their lives with me over the years. I hope they find this book useful, if not enjoyable.

I wish to thank the publishers for granting permission to reprint parts of the following:

'Revisioning women and drug use: gender sensitivity, gendered bodies and reducing harm', *International Journal of Drugs Policy*, 15, 5–6 (2004): 327–35.

Thanks go to Jill Lake, my editor at Palgrave for her kind advice, and to Andee Rudloff for letting me use one of her lovely designs for the book cover. And to Imma, of course, with whom I celebrated my civil partnership during the writing of this book, my deepest gratitude.

Elizabeth Ettorre

1
The 'Back Story' on Women, Drugs and the Body

> From the time when Florence Nightingale was called a camp follower up to the present day . . . the battle of the sexes has been waged in the most inappropriate arena I can imagine: the centers of healing . . .
>
> Miriam Gilbert (1970: 62)

Changing the world for women drug users

This introduction is all about providing the 'back story' for how *Revisioning women and drug use* emerged. It's almost as if this book has its own life and personal history. *Revisioning women and drug use* has been a long time coming and represents for me an overwhelming research journey from despair to hope as my body moved from being ill to healthy (see Ettorre, 2005a). Because of this experience, I learned a greater sense of compassion and empathy towards women drug users' quest for well-being, while at the same time personifying polluted bodies or living symbols of degraded women. Although I am not a drug-using woman, I feel passionately about women who use drugs and I want this book to speak to them and to their needs. My illness experience has taught me humility.

With the above ideas in mind, I would like to set into motion a debate about how we can move forward in our field. In order to move forward, we have to build upon our past. I don't think it is particularly useful if we discard everything in our past and begin all over again from scratch. Rather we need to choose deliberately how we will transform our knowledge, paradigms, discourses, notions and practices which are capable of being transformed. Hence, we need to 'revision', which means letting go of how we have seen in order to construct new perceptions (Clarke and Olesen, 1999: 3). We need to let go of our damaging, prejudicial, unjust, outdated images and ideas about drug users, particularly women drug users, in order to construct new insights and theories about their drug-using experiences. It is my hope that my focus on revisioning will make this book quite distinctive in focus.

Also, to place the book into perspective for the reader is to make you aware that this book is primarily a theoretical piece. However, while it is not based upon an empirical study of women, drugs and the body, it offers more than knowledge and data from observations, surveys, clinical trials, and so on. Given that theory based on women drug users' experience should be indispensable in this field (Ettorre, 2004), I took a different and needed tack: to focus my energy on developing theory derived from experience, accessible and reflexive, and subject to revision in light of experience (Stanley and Wise, 1990: 24) – women's experiences. In effect, I did an intensive literature search and review of articles, reports and books published on women and drugs in Europe, Australia and North America from 1995 until 2005. Using these secondary sources as the foundation for my data is a strategy similar to the one I used in my earlier work (Ettorre, 1992). I believe this type of strategy for the current book can be successful in illuminating emergent issues on gender, drugs and the body.

Over the years, my desire to develop theory in the drugs field has grown. I believe that as a researcher and theoretician, I am able to be on the same critical plane as my subjects of study, women drug users. Accordingly, I want to appear as a 'real historical individual' with concrete, specific desires and interests (Harding 1987a: 9). As this historical individual, I am a researcher and theoretician committed to a political position in which knowledge is defined altruistically as 'knowledge for' (Stanley, 1990: 15) and where I am able to develop a sharp focus on the concepts of difference, intersectionality and multiplicity (Moosa-Mitha 2004: 63). For me, this is a viable and visible position in which I attempt to see the notion of difference as multidimensional and theorize difference with regard to multiple levels of analysis.

I want not only to create new ideas but also to help change the world for women drug users. This may appear at first glance a grandiose or naïve claim. Nevertheless, it is true. I want to begin by helping to create a society which is 'difference centred' and which acknowledges the marginality of drug users, specifically drug-using women. I want to cast doubt on normative beliefs and practices that are shaped in both marginalized and privileged spaces. I want to make those who hold these normative beliefs feel uncomfortable. The whole point of my doing this work is not only to make observations and theories but also to affect changes that are structural, relational and cultural. My underlying logic is that theorization is yet another site of struggling against oppression (Moosa-Mitha 2004: 63).

As I continue to provide this book's back story, I will divide this first chapter into four interrelated discussions. First, I will discuss briefly what I call my anti-oppressive research journey and how this journey relates to the aims of this book. Second, I look at the tensions that exist in our field between gender viewed as a quirk and gender viewed as a key to understanding drug cultures. (I will discuss gender as a theoretical notion more generally in the following chapter.) Third, I want to examine two co-existing paradigms, the 'classical' and the 'postmodern', and compare and contrast them. In the concluding section, I look at the remaining structure of the book and ask, 'Where do we go from here?'

Taking an anti-oppressive research journey

Revisioning women and drug use has been a veritable research journey. I have 'visited' a plethora of studies carried out on women drug users in a variety of relevant areas. In my journey, I have been searching for work which offers anti-oppressive approaches to the women drug users we study. I must admit that I have been rather disappointed. In this journey, I have found few authors who offer approaches which challenge the status quo. So, I begin this book with the clear assumption that not only theoretical but also critical work on women and drug use is urgently needed if we are to offer emancipatory or liberatory approaches in the drugs field. I firmly believe that these types of approaches are the only ones which propose social justice for women and other drug users. Why are we doing this work anyway, if not to help those we research?

Given that women drug users live on the margins of many, if not all societies, these women, similar to all people who live their lives on the margins, experience silencing and injustice (Kovach, 2005: 21). We need to ensure that we make our research political merely on the basis of who these drug-using women are. I wrote this book with the desire to be 'political' and challenge the sorts of epistemologies and methodologies which dominate the drugs field. More importantly, these epistemologies and methodologies have the effect of dehumanizing and depersonalizing those on the margins. They also justify social injustice and inequalities on the basis of differences from the ideal white, heterosexual, male, Enlightened subject (Strega, 2004: 215). In achieving this aim, I attempt to draw together empirical studies on women and drug use and offer a comprehensive analysis of gendered bodies and drug use. I want to examine our drug-using society with regard to its implications for social inequality, injustice and exclusion and the governing mentalities (Campbell, 2000) of power, gender, embodiment and risk. In fulfilling these aims, I endeavour to offer a fresh approach, as well as 'transgressive possibilities' (Brown and Strega, 2004: 1) for us as researchers in the drugs field.

Here I contend that the complexities of the development of ideas around power, gender, embodiment and risk are instructive for scholars in the drugs field and should help to inform feminist approaches. Already in earlier work (Ettorre 1992; Ettorre and Riska, 1995) I have argued for the need for gender sensitivity in the drugs field, and along with others (see Measham, 2002; Evans et al., 2002; Raine, 2001; Murphy and Rosenbaum, 1999; Sterk, 1999; Boyd, 1999; Henderson, 1996; Anderson, 1995), I argue that gender sensitivity is still lacking in this field. At this point, I want to emphasize the 'F' word, feminism. In my view, feminist ways of thinking are not passé or outdated within the academy. Indeed, feminist ideas have had a significant impact on the academy (Farnham, 1987) and continue to do so – no matter what colleagues both academic or not may say. Nevertheless, there has been a strong backlash which has returned gender to sex, making social inequalities disappear inside the body (Oakley, 1997: 34). This has been helped along by academic feminism's becoming lost in a fog of social constructionism (Oakley, 1997: 42).

However, a major problem has been the ways in which education and research, including feminism, are used as weapons of colonialization (Rich, 1980; Humm, 1992) and confirmation of Western ways of thinking. In the 'academic' arena of the drugs field, feminism has never been taken very seriously nor considered as a viable research concern or option. In our field, biomedical and criminal justice models predominate, while the masculinist focus of these models is not only highly visible but also rigidly adhered to. Within a masculinist focus, the belief is that women have actually made it; their struggles for liberation or at least equality are over and 'women' are now incorporated into majority culture. Usually those who hold these sorts of misplaced views do not attempt to expand their ways of thinking to include women at the margins, including Black and ethnic minority women, transgender and lesbian women, indigenous women, disabled women, and so on. It is my view that until social justice is attained for *all* women, both those at the centre and on the margins, feminism is still needed as a form of embodied, intellectual and political resistance. This is why in *Revisioning women and drug use* I want to build upon contemporary feminist ways of thinking alongside emancipatory, anti-oppressive and liberatory approaches. In taking a step, albeit small, in that direction I seek to challenge the overwhelming masculinist focus in the academic area of the drugs field.

Although I tend to use the concept of gender quite a lot in this book, this use is not meant to imply that I have forgotten the concept 'women'. On the contrary, maintaining a feminist perspective which acknowledges that women, especially marginal women, are silenced and devalued is central to my way of thinking. Of course, I want to avoid essentializing women or perpetuating the idea that all women are the same, a homogeneous group. Still, with special reference to drugs use, I would like to contextualize the oppressive dynamics that shape the world through the lens of the ideal white, heterosexual, male, Enlightenment point of view.

Gender – an imperative in understanding drug cultures

When I first started working in the drugs field in the 1970s, women drug users were hidden from view. They were marginalized and stigmatized, while being silenced and the targets of social injustice. To mark 1975 as the International Year of Women, Orianna Josseau Kalant edited a now classic text, *Alcohol and drug problems in women*. In her Introduction, she argued that research on women and substance misuse was a 'non-field'. She stated quite openly in making this now well-quoted statement that the subjects of choice in addiction research areas were most frequently males, ranging from rats to college students (Kalant, 1980: 1). Her point was not to replace male with female rats or male with female college students in research designs or scientific investigations. Rather, Kalant was capitalizing on how sex differences tended to be overlooked and this was, as she said, extremely frustrating.

Almost thirty years on, it is still extremely wearisome because in comparison to studies of men and drug use, studies of women and drug use remain relatively rare (South and Teeman, 1999). Indeed, studies like Rosenbaum's classic *Women on heroin* (1981) stand in 'splendid isolation' (Pearson, 1999a: 482). Despite an increase in gender-related research and research comparing gender differences, women have remained 'the second sex' in diagnostic definition, theory development and clinical trial involvement (Stein and Cyr, 1997: 993). This 'empiricist' type of work is qualitatively different from in-depth, exploratory studies of female drug users (see, for example, Friedman and Alicea, 2001) which expose a sympathetic, if not empathetic position.

This long-established resistance to gender sensitive or feminist approaches by researchers in the drugs field (Ettorre, 1992) will hopefully break down in future. While amongst researchers there is an easy acceptance of gender as a researcher's whim or a quirk in the drug world, it is more difficult to acknowledge the centrality of gender in the lives of women drug users. In this context, contemporary work that draws attention to the intricacies of gender (Raine, 2001) and underscores how within the gendered environment of drug use, women 'do drugs' differently from men (Measham, 2002) has been promising. Undeniably, work carried out within the past decade accentuates the importance of gender-sensitive and/or feminist perspectives for treatment and policy (Kandall, 1996; Stevens and Wexler, 1998; Sterk, 1999; Klee, Jackson and Lewis, 2001; Raine, 2001; Friedman and Alicea, 2001) and developments on the level of theory (Irwin, 1995; Boyd, 1999; Campbell, 1999, 2000; Denton and O'Malley, 1999; Henderson, 1999; Murphy and Rosenbaum, 1999; Wright, 2002; Evans, Forsyth and Gauthier, 2002; Hunt, Joe-Laidler and Evans, 2002; Measham, 2002). Clearly if gender is of pivotal importance to our understanding of drug cultures (Measham, 2002), there appears to be a tension in our recognition of the wide-ranging significance of gender in the field.

Two co-existing paradigms

In delving into the above-mentioned tension in our knowledge of the overall significance of gender and drugs, I am keen to flag up key notions and related research practices that characterize two simultaneous paradigms of drug use: the 'classical' and 'postmodern'. I contend that the latter is more gender sensitive and conducive to feminist, emancipatory and anti-oppressive stances, while the former is rather obsolete. Let us now look critically at these two paradigms.

Classical paradigm

The classical paradigm concentrates on disease-related aspects of drug use and misuse. Experts, whether researchers, policy-makers or clinicians, focus on the spread of the disease, addiction. While these experts tend to use individualistic, causal explanations, their level of analysis tends to be on the 'sick' individual rather than communities or society. Nevertheless, universalizing statements are often made, reflecting the view that drugs are inherently evil, and their use undermines individual health and leads to the disintegration of community and society (Coomber and South, 2004a: 13–14). In particular, drug use is supposed to lead to or cause anti-social behaviour, if not serious crime. Drugs are expected to make people do treacherous things, justifying overwhelming criminal responses.

Within this paradigm, numerous stereotypes and myths such as the myth of addiction (Hammersley and Reid, 2002: 13) based on exaggeration and distortion of the effects of drugs are upheld because they are viewed as 'socially functional' for a wide range of groups. In this context, illegal actors such as those involved in the production and trafficking of controlled drugs have their prices go up. Or others, such as drug users themselves, get convenient explanations for their drug use and become an everyday part of drug folklore. Ex-drug users replace addiction to drugs with addiction to groups against drugs as they are seen to re-integrate into society (Hammersley and Reid, 2002: 14). With regard to the social functionality of 'legal' social actors, such as those connected to the police, customs and excise, the pharmaceutical business, the white-dominated male press, religious and moral groups, they benefit as responses to drug use become a veritable 'industry'. In this process gender issues are made invisible, naturalized or reduced to complicated brain processes (Reid and Hammersley, 2000: 171). (See, for example, Jellinek (1960); Valliant (1973); Edwards et al., (1976); and Plant (1981).)

Psychiatrists and other mental health specialists have had a major hand in confirming this idea of addiction and in turn have developed an epidemiological focus (Edwards, 1978) and more recently, an ecological model (Edwards, 2004) which privileges disease and intervention systems, respectively. Their 'thank you theory' operates on the basis that when the patient is cured he or she will thank the therapist, even though the patient was an unwilling participant (Bean, 2004: 231). Psychiatrists are the key biomedical players in the environment of treatment, intervention and prevention of drug use, although in recent years the cadre of workers in the drugs field has included more non-clinical specialists who embody a psychiatric mentality. This is because the tier of non-substance misuse treatment services that interfaces with drug treatment services has been identified and developed (Hayes, 2004: 215).

Within the classical paradigm, grand theories or narratives explaining drug use as deviant behaviour, behaviour that stigmatizes and marginalizes users, exist (van Wormer and Davis, 2003: 50). Undeniably, drug users are morally reprimanded and culturally disciplined. They have the 'disease of addiction' that is somehow embedded in their bodies (de Belleroche, 2002) or perhaps genetic as other substance misuse such as alcohol apparently is (Peters and Preedy, 2002). Even if social and cultural factors are taken into account, these factors are presented in a deterministic way as a part of 'neurobiological fine tuning' (Hill, 2000: 461).

'Hegemonic' moral panics (McRobbie and Thorton, 1995) emerging from positions of privilege are generated by the media to remind the entire population of drug users' deviance and to separate these 'timewasters' or 'social malingerers' from the mainstream. Whether or not 'Wars on drugs' are media-stimulated, 'armistices' appear to redefine the boundaries of containment, surveillance and control (Ben-Yehuda, 1994). 'Armistices' mean that another, different group of drugs users may have their passports confiscated by the powers that be or that punitive strategies are used to keep drug users in line by arresting their treaters as in the Wintercomfort case in Cambridge, England (Shapiro, 2000; Flemen, 2004).

Here the notions of intersectionality or anti-oppressive are alien conceptions, as a Western ethnocentric view of drug use prevails (Coomber and South, 2004a: 14). Indeed, issues such as race, ethnicity, class, gender and age tend to be overlooked because most experts are interested in maintaining the hegemony of the 'West over the rest' (Littlewood, 2002). Middle class, young, White, male, Western concerns take priority over other ones in this monolithic perspective (Coomber and South, 2004a: 15). No one questions the incarceration of women offenders, the grave impact that this has on poor women of colour or that in the United States the proportion of African American females who are incarcerated is seven times higher than for White females (Roberts, Jackson and Carlton-Laney, 2000: 903). Additionally, there is no conception of disability – it is believed that drug use is a drug user's main disability and that this disability is a moral one. If you are a disabled person and you can't walk, see or hear, you have an even more difficult time as a drug user (Li, Ford and Moore, 2000) being or having been most probably a victim of violence.

In the classical paradigm, there is a tendency to 'treat' single substances within a hierarchy of drugs (Ettorre, 1992). Abstinence (Westermeyer and Boedicker, 2000; Mertens and Weisner, 2001), not harm reduction is the key issue in rehabilitating users and bringing them back to 'society's fold'. Prohibition is the ultimate goal. If harm minimization is mentioned it is usually referring to the minimization of harm to the community rather than the individual user (Berridge, 1998:102). In this paradigm, drug users appear to have 'rights' only if they stop using drugs: their 'welfare takes precedence over their wants' (Seedhouse, 1998: 192–3).

Only ex-users have rights and these are somewhat limited (Smart, 1984). Women users appear to have fewer rights than men, especially if they are expectant mothers (Murphy and Rosenbaum, 1999). Given that the governing mentality or cultural production of ideas and images related to illegal drugs (Campbell, 1999) of the classical paradigm is masculinist to its very core, an 'ideology of sacred maternity that sacralizes motherhood at the expense of women's subjectivity' (Klassen, 2001: 775) is rampant and targets pregnant drug users.

Postmodern paradigm

Alongside the classical paradigm is what I call the postmodern paradigm. (See for example, Waldorf et al., 1991; Ettorre, 1992; Parker et al., 1998; South, 1999; Murphy and Rosenbaum, 1999; Measham et al., 2001; Monaghan, 2001; Measham, 2002; Parker, Williams and Aldridge, 2002; Coomber and South, 2004b.) Within the postmodern paradigm, more useful ideas and concerns have arisen than in the classical one because not only does this paradigm deal more success-fully with standard, persistent notions of inequality, such as race, class and gender, and so on, but also this paradigm paves the way for an anti-oppressive approach. Plainly, the importance of 'context' is appreciated (Coomber and South, 2004a). Here the level of analysis tends to be on the collective and social rather than the individual. No one discipline dominates this paradigm: the quest for under-standing appears interdisciplinary and developing cultural and social awareness is viewed as crucial.

Most, if not all social scientists working within this paradigm would agree that rituals can unite people into a community and that celebratory rituals are normal, as is taking mind altering substances (Douglas, 1987: 4). The importance of understanding rituals tends to take precedence over using stereotypes and upholding social myths. Rituals are viewed as scripted performative moments and enactments of embodied identities (Langman, 2003: 225). In this context, women drug users may share an enthusiasm for the acute effects of drugs (Erickson et al., 2000: 773). However, in these performative moments and enactments of their embodied identities, women drug users can be seen to enact pleasure side by side with negative emotions and 'dis-pleasure'. Also, intersectionality becomes possible within this paradigm as the importance of developing approaches based on social differences such as race, class and gender are recognized and valued. Here difference is treated as the foundation of exclusion rather than an exclusionary position. Difference in itself is privileged as a theoret-ical category, a site of political practice and an enactment of human rights. All drug users have human rights that are not contingent on whether or not they stop using drugs.

Thus the postmodern paradigm begins to deal with ethics and the basic human rights of drug users (Ettorre 1992: 57). Moral panics are replaced by conscious awareness and subsequent conceptual movements to a more participatory and relational view of bearing witness to the social injustices that drug users face. These conceptual movements allow for the experience of drug use to be transformed into a testimonial project of everyday discrimination. Here testimony to drug users is able to emerge as a dialogical form of address. Simply, this requires attentive and ethical forms of listening (Ahmed and Stacey, 2001: 6) from those around drug users.

Moreover this paradigm focuses on drug use as a social issue that is culturally shaped into a social problem and reflective of 'disreputable pleasures' (O'Malley and Valverde, 2004). Professional experts are needed as much as drug users themselves. They are the lay experts who have a voice because they experience drug use and the problems related to it. Drug users are also seen as the consumers of drugs that become intertwined with the cultures of everyday life (Ruggiero, 1999). Here, theorists critical of a 'war on drugs' note that what was once a largely innocuous, consensual, consumer market has been transformed into what is routinely described in policy terms as a war zone (Pearson, 1999a: 478).

Consumption cultures are poly-drug cultures where users may or may not consume their drugs of choice, but at least they consume a substance that makes them feel high or provides psychotropic effects. Parker and Measham (1994) call this the 'pick 'n' mix' scene. In this paradigm, proponents recognize that this realm of consumer culture in contemporary society is a site for the reproduction of social inequalities and a fortification of normativity. Consumption of drugs flourishes within a society 'addicted itself to the sorry tension between individual excess and social control' (Ferrel and Sanders, 1995: 313). These drug cultures have a particular impact on young people (Ettorre and Miles, 2001), given that their lives are all about occupying distinct social spaces in the routes of consumption, reproduction and production, all of which are located in specific gender, sex, class and race contexts (Griffin, 1997). Furthermore the policing of drug consumption and the role of schools in policing drugs' impact on young people's perceptions of drug consumption is a risky business in an environment where the availability of drugs is a normal part of the 'leisure-pleasure landscape' (Parker et al., 1995: 25).

Rather than grand theories, local narratives of normalization are constructed with a reconsideration of the subject, object and author of research. These narratives focusing on consumers or users with specific needs and demands may conflict with local policies of containment and control, shaped by surveillance systems such as the police, customs and social services. In this context, community-based services within the context of multi-agency responses become the order of the day (Teeman, South and Henderson, 1999). There is also space for the development of Afrocentric treatment principles (Roberts, Jackson and Carlton-Laney, 2000: 903) or treatments sensitive to indigenous people (Segal, 2001). In particular for women a holistic approach which addresses relationship dynamics, communication skills, assertiveness and vocational skills becomes a real possibility in this way of thinking (Sterk, Elifson and Theall, 2000).

Within this paradigm, drug users may be transgressors but only in so far as their rule breaking is part and parcel of being poor, unemployed, homeless, victims and/or perpetrators of violence. Thus, social exclusion is viewed as a key factor in shaping the transgression of drug use (Pearson, 1999b). In this paradigm, safer sex and harm minimization strategies are catchwords as well as practices that aware users will exploit with their significant others, within their peer groups and/or in public, rave, dance or consumer settings.

To my mind, the postmodern paradigm appears the most responsive to social inequalities because of its fluid, discursive methods and expansive scope as regards all things social and cultural. Within this paradigm, there are recognisable 'bio-struggles' in which individuals such as drug users attempt to break from the clutch of governing mentalities (Campbell, 2000) and disciplinary powers *vis-à-vis* drug use. These bio-struggles unleash the development of new bodies and pleasures which have the potential to undermine the construction of normalized subjects (Best and Kellner, 1991: 58). Regardless of this radical deployment of bodies, a postmodern paradigm should include within its epistemological focus a vision of the future which does not: (i) deconstruct or debase gender as an issue (Maynard, 1994:19), nor (ii) deny that 'subjugated knowledges' can be an important part of transforming our social worlds (Harding, 1987b: 188–9).

These two paradigms, the classic and the postmodern, co-exist in the drugs field today. At times, the differences between them which were outlined above may not appear in such a sharp contrast. However, general tendencies do appear. Given that I do not want to create binary opposites, I want to emphasize that, in the main, they represent two general bodies of thinking or paradigms which have emerged over the years in the drugs field. Sometimes, they overlap, sometimes they diverge and sometimes they contradict each other. Nevertheless I would contend that the postmodern paradigm is more humane than the classical given that the voices of drug users tend to be heard rather than silenced and furthermore, social inequalities, in particular class, gender, race and ethnic ones, are more readily acknowledged. Most importantly, difference is able to become a clear theoretical category, as well as a site of resistance.

In this book, I aim to develop my ideas from within a postmodern paradigm and I hope that I will be able to maintain throughout an anti-oppressive stance from within this perspective. I don't want to have my head in the clouds, so to speak, and use words that will alienate the reader. I want to be clear headed and offer to you, the reader, some novel conceptions. It is my hope that, by building upon the benefits of postmodern paradigms, I will be able to develop existing ideas about gender further and introduce the body as a central concept within this paradigm which I see as being friendly to a feminist embodiment approach. As a drug researcher I want in this book to explore specifically issues that are central to women in this area, as well as the overall impact of the notion of embodiment on drug use. Thus, I will examine both empirical data and theories on drug use through the dual lens of gender and the body.

Accordingly the discussions in this book should provide an excellent opportunity to develop and extend theories of drug use which continue to marginalize drug users, especially women. Mainly, illegal drug use will be considered but reference will be made to the hierarchy of both legal and illegal drugs. Gender will be explored as both a complex social process and an established cultural institution or regulatory regime (see the following chapter). The governing mentality (Campbell, 2000) in the drugs discourse remains that women should not take drugs and work in the field reflects this mentality, regardless of the emergence of 'designer drugs' or the apparent 'feminization' of drugs such as ecstasy (Henderson, 1993; 1999). Gendering processes, as well as the governing mentalities (Campbell, 2000) about women drug users are institutionalizing processes which are having wide-ranging social effects. As sensitive researchers we should be aware of these damaging effects, particularly on those we study.

Where do we go from here?

With the above ideas in mind, I want the discussions in the following chapters to construct an anti-oppressive, feminist embodiment approach to drug use – an approach which translates some of the feminist thinking around bodies and embodiment into our field. Specifically, in the following chapter, 'Feminist theorizing about drugs: gender, power and the body', I begin to construct this sort of approach. I outline the key notions of gender, embodiment and power and link them to those social theorists who employ them in their theoretical work. The concept 'embodied deviance' is introduced and linked with the four bodily tasks of restraint, reproduction, representation and regulation. I attempt in this chapter not only to lay the groundwork for a feminist embodiment approach to women and drugs but also to demonstrate that a clear understanding of key embodiment issues in the experiences of women drug users needs to become visible in the drugs field, if we are to move on.

In Chapter 3, 'Punishing or privileging marginalization?', I continue the task of developing a feminist embodied approach to drugs by analysing additional notions related to women drug users through the lens of the lived body. These notions are pollution, dependence, cultures of emotions and pleasure. Again, as in the previous chapter, I contend that these are key notions. I argue that they provide more conceptual armaments in developing a feminist embodiment theory on drugs; help us to foster a view from the margins; allow us to favour subjugated knowledge about women and drugs; and help us to transform the conditions of women drug users' lives.

In Chapter 4, 'Embodying core activities: gendered perfomativities', I take a close look at Tammy Anderson's (2005) novel ideas on women drug users' 'core activities' in the illegal drugs world. In this chapter, I continue feminist theorizing by establishing additional theoretical links with her work and maintaining an intense focus on the female body. Thus I look closely at the effects of Anderson's core activities on women's drug-using bodies. How these core activities or dimensions of women's power in the illicit drug economy can be conceptualized as 'embodied' caring work is my main concern in this chapter. I also offer a brief critique of Anderson's views and argue why an embodiment perspective is a necessary corrective to what she offers.

In Chapters 5 through to 7, I look specifically at how gendered, 'real bodies' (Evans and Lee, 2002) become visible in the drugs field as historically and culturally specific and how these bodies need both social and individual affirmation. In each of the three chapters I look at specific contexts and situations with special reference to gendered embodiment. I ask, 'How can we develop a feminist embodiment approach to drug use?' and subsequently detail some of the different types of embodiments that are on offer to drug-using women.

Specifically, in Chapter 5, 'Drug-consuming bodies', I attempt to embed the notion of consuming bodies in the contemporary material culture of illegal drugs. I examine the sociological field of consumption and review features of modern consumer culture with regard to drug-consuming bodies. I do this by drawing upon the work of contemporary sociologists who have written theoretically about consumption. Distinctive characteristics of contemporary consumer culture, the relationship between urbanization and consumption, the body in consumer culture and 'consumption themes' are all outlined with special reference to drug consumption. I attempt to weave together these ideas within an anti-oppressive, feminist embodiment perspective and emphasize the need to consider the ordinariness of drug consumption for some, if not most users.

Focusing on the regulatory regime of reproduction in which a range of disciplinary practices target pregnant bodies, I look closely in Chapter 6 at 'Drug-using reproducing bodies'. I envisage these as the 'real' material sites (that is, gendered bodies) upon which the chaos and disorder of drug use are inscribed. I look at these bodies as part and parcel of the somatic society and how drug-using pregnant bodies are visualized through the 'scopic drive', a characteristic of this type of society. I contend that pregnant drug-using bodies are material sites related to the culturally constructed notion of 'disordered body'. The belief that the pregnant drug-using body is shaped as a deviant body, separated from other female bodies, is examined.

Chapter 7, 'Contaminated drug-using bodies', offers a fresh approach to HIV/AIDS and injecting drug use with special reference to female embodiment. In this chapter I challenge the idea that drug users are material conduits of HIV/AIDS. Also, the false belief which has emerged in the public's consciousness that HIV/AIDS is a treatable disease is examined as a type of dangerous normalization bolstered by racism. In this context, I build up this fresh approach to HIV/AIDS and injecting drug use by examining the masculinist concerns in this area; women's functionality *vis-à-vis* heterosexuality and the traditional link between prostitution and drug use, or what I call the 'whore, drugs and risk cultural configuration'. I also look critically at women drug users' bodies in the postmodern moment of HIV/AIDS. This chapter is a real attempt to distinguish different discourses organizing the expression of the embodied experience of women injecting drug users confronting HIV/AIDS.

These chapters are followed by the concluding chapter, Chapter 8, 'Embodiment, emotions and female drug use', in which I look at the affective dimensions of gendered drug use and examine emotions side by side women's drug-using bodies. I consider how emotions have a crucial part to play in the morality of gendered, drug-using bodies and ask a series of key questions. These questions are related to how the emotional economy of women drug users becomes embodied; how the consensus on emotions by those who study emotions connects to the affective embodiment of women drug users; the affective dimensions of risk as culturally dependent embodied processes and types of feminist strategies needed for women drug users to achieve successful embodiment. Hopefully, the reader will become aware that there is a need for broader conceptions of women and drug use which move us onto the terrain of embodiment. We need approaches to women and drug use that are grounded in the material sites of our bodies as these material entities become shaped by race, class, culture, age, sexual orientation and able-bodiedness. Most importantly, we need theories which no longer repress the body or passion in our ways of thinking (Gatens, 1992: 135).

2
Feminist Theorizing about Drugs: Gender, Power and the Body

> With the rise of modern feminism an inquiry into the nature of women was undertaken, for the first time by women themselves. It is no wonder that we cannot agree on what we find. As soon as we stopped seeing ourselves as Freud saw us, as people who do not possess penises, disagreement began . . .
>
> Signe, Hammer (1975: 3)

Surfacing of the body

In the previous chapter, we became familiar with the 'back story' for the development of this book. I suggested that gender may be viewed as a fanciful quirk in our analyses of the lives of drug users or as a crucial notion in our understanding of drug cultures. Additionally, I presented two co-existing paradigms, the 'classical and the 'postmodern', and suggested that the latter is more conducive to the study of gender, as well as an anti-oppressive way of thinking. While there is arguably a need for approaches and perspectives on addiction and drug use that highlight the complexities of gender (Raine, 2001), the concept of gender needs to be recognized as a fundamental one in the drugs field. With this awareness, I do not want in the current chapter to construct a 'story' of how gender systems are constructed and maintained in the drugs field or how these become systems of domination or oppressive to women drug users. I take for granted that these systems exist and how easily they become embedded in the everyday lives of drug users, as well as research and clinical practice. Rather I want to revision the issue of women and drugs in a fresh light by exploring the theoretical links between gender, power and the body.

Within the history of the social sciences, the surfacing of the body as a key theoretical site is a relatively recent occurrence (Turner, 1996). Specifically, 'second wave' feminists' efforts in the realm of women's health attracted feminist social science scholars during the 1970s and cleared the way for the development of the body as a vital theoretical notion (Davis, 1997: 4). While the body has become the site for the life project within late modernity, bodies are cultural and social beings – fleshy and 'boned' entities where we inscribe normalized, as well as stigmatized identities. The body is a central point for struggles over power: a foundation of social identities which are inscribed upon our social, relational and corporeal lives. In this context, drug cultures are not only gendered, body cultures but also spaces where the female body emerges as a site for the commonplace acts of contestation, resistance and rebellion, as well as conformity. This 'dirtied' or polluted gendered body becomes a metaphor for *failed* femininity, emotionality, sexuality and a breakdown of self-risk management (Malloch, 2004). (See the following chapter and Chapter 7 for a discussion of the notion of polluted and contaminated bodies.)

The current chapter is divided into three main discussions. First, I take the initial step of constructing a feminist embodiment perspective on women and drugs by defining the three key notions of gender, embodiment and power. Second, I outline the work of selected theorists who operationalize these respective notions in their work and hopefully demonstrate the need for feminist embodiment theories on drugs. In the concluding part of the chapter, the gendered body culture of the drug-using world is examined by using the concept 'embodied deviance' in relation to the four bodily tasks of restraint, reproduction, representation and regulation.

Two assumptions run throughout this chapter: (i) a postmodern paradigm facilitates the development of feminist embodiment theories on drugs use, as suggested earlier, and (ii) a clear understanding of key embodiment issues in the experiences of women drug users needs to become visible in the drugs field. This assumption is based on the goal of feminist theory – the fact that we consider gender as our central subject (Flax, 1990: 21). Here, by exploring the complex links between gender, the body and power, I hope to offer a cogent understanding of the contested character of the cultural representations of female drug use. I want to build up an appreciation of responsive explorations of the complex ways in which gender and drug use come together and how this appreciation is achievable on a collective level for women drug users. Additionally, I hope to challenge the status quo.

Building a feminist embodiment perspective

In the previous chapter, when I clarified the differences between the classical and postmodern paradigms in the drugs field, I suggested that a clear benefit of a postmodern paradigm is its fluid method and expansive scope to include all things social and cultural. That the postmodern paradigm is more adaptable to contemporary society and the rapid cultural transformations that we experience is central. More importantly, in a postmodern paradigm theorists develop conceptions of social criticism which do not rely on traditional, one-dimensional philosophical underpinnings: legitimation of ideas becomes plural, local and immanent (Fraser and Nicolson, 1990: 21–23). In my view, a postmodern paradigm develops workable ideas on gender and embodiment and a thorough understanding of both concepts, gender and the body, and enhances our insights into women drug users' lives. Their lives begin to appear as multidimensional, as well as full of human, social intricacies.

While gender is a contested concept within the postmodern paradigm, its proponents recognize the tension between the preservation of gender consciousness and identity as a source of political unity, as well as alternative visions and the destruction of gender prescriptions which limit human choice and possibility (Bordo, 1990: 153). Thus, given that it is becoming increasingly difficult to think of the world ordered from the vantage point of one woman, the ontological conceit of the Western, female subject (that is, White woman) becomes untenable (Probyn, 1990: 177). In the following discussions I summarize my ideas on gender and embodiment and include my thinking on the notion of power, which I view as essential in developing these ideas. I will then look at 'gender sensitive', if not feminist theories of embodiment and make links with the drugs field.

Gender as a social process and regulatory regime

Within a postmodern paradigm, gender is all about the powerful shaping of our bodies along the narrow constraints of sexual differences. Consistent with this paradigm are explorations by feminist sociologists who view gender as both a process and a regulatory regime or a cultural institution (Lorber, 1994). As a process, gender is part of all human interactions. It is relational, cultural and social. It is characterized by repetitive, regulatory practices which mould the meaning of 'female' and 'male' and 'masculinity' and 'femininity' on the cultural, political and economic levels. Gender can be seen to have an effect on the social groupings of men and women; sentient bodies being 'naturalized' into one sex or another and divisions between both the private and the public arenas of our social lives. Gender brings to society a set of regulatory practices centred on the performance of normality, while individual bodies are marked by differences on the basis of being male and female, as well as masculine and feminine. In effect, gender requires and institutes its own distinctive regulatory and disciplinary regime (Butler, 2004: 41).

As a regulatory regime or an institution, gender is a part of culture. It is similar to other components of culture such as symbols, language, mores, norms, values and so on. Gender is a discursive form of fragile, yet structured social inequality and it is embedded in our cultures. Nevertheless, the differences on which gender identities are marshalled are continually being undermined so that the field of popular culture comprises a to and fro movement between the doing and undoing of gender (McRobbie, 2005: 71). This means that while gender is a normative, moralizing discursive regime that exerts social control on all people in society, its boundaries are constantly being shifted and redefined.

But gender differences also intersect with other forms of social inequality, such as class, race and ethnicity and these intersections compound our experiences of gender. Within a Butlerian (1993, 1990) context, gender's performativity is important as a practice of coercion, a forceful shaping of bodies along the narrow constraints of gender differences (McRobbie, 2005: 84). This exposes the importance of analysing gender's disciplinary and regulatory practices as well as the possibilities of flexibility and change issuing from these practices. Given the above, feminist 'gender' work provides a clear steer on gender's embeddedness in the social lives of drug users.

In the drugs field, proponents of the postmodern paradigm such as Hunt et al. (2002), Measham (2002), Evans et al. (2002), Irwin (1995), Campbell (1999; 2000), and so on appreciate the importance of gender and gender relationships. Their appreciation is based on recognizing the complexities of gender as a process and a regulatory regime. Then again, if gender was truly accepted as a process and regulatory regime or social institution, we would no longer need to direct our attention specifically towards these issues. We would no longer need 'special' work (Raine, 2001; Boyd, 1999; Ettorre, 1992) concentrating on women drug users. We would recognize the subtle and often hidden and unanticipated ways that gender permeates all areas of the lives of drug users – both men and women. The fact that researchers found that heroin may be a source of male, street, cultural capital (Collison, 1996) and ecstasy transformed women into 'divas' in the dance scene (Henderson, 1996) are important gender issues. These studies reveal how gender can be used as a template for gathering important knowledge on drug use. However, I would still contend that we have little information on how gender as a process and an institution influences the ways in which users coordinate their space, their place, their time, their drugs management, their community resources and their relationships with significant others, whether these others be other drug users, relatives, families, treaters, and so on. Access to drugs, knowledge of drugs, use of drugs and help for misuse of drugs – all involve hidden and sometimes not so hidden gendered processes.

For example, in relevant, topical work (Ettorre and Riska, 1995, 2001; Riska and Ettorre, 1999), psychotropic drug users (that is, those using both minor and major tranquillisers) were marked as drug users, albeit legal ones, who feel their 'nerves' and somatize their 'stress'. We found that experiences of psychotropic use and misuse differ for men and women users and we identified 'feminized nerves' and 'masculinized stress' in that prior empirical study. Why do psycho-tropic drug users contextualize their experiences in gendered ways? Why are the sources of women's problems with psychotropic drugs linked to their private, emotional and/or relational lives and men's with their external work lives? Why are physicians more willing to support men stopping these drugs than women? The answers to all of these questions went beyond our research. But they reveal that unambiguous gendered expectations, gendered norms, gendered styles and gendered rules of engagement exist in the drugs world and that these gender issues are not easy to uncover.

Traditionally, in drug cultures what is male or characterized as masculine takes priority over what is female or characterized as feminine (Perry, 1979), a prioritization of the cultural machinations of gender. Gender is embedded in our drug-using cultures and treatment systems and not taking gender seriously can have major health implications (Brettevillejensen, 1999; Brunswick and Messeri, 1999; Chitwood et al., 2001; Abercrombie and Booth, 1997). Additionally, while drug treatment systems were designed originally for men (Vogt, 1998), that is not a good enough reason to argue that this is why treatment systems have been slow to change their methods to meet the needs of women. Here I am not speaking about intellectual advancement. I am speaking about meeting the basic human rights of drug users. We need to recognize that these rights themselves are gendered and that drug policies which do not explicitly acknowledge these inalienable rights, particularly women's rights, may have adverse consequences (Campbell, 1999: 900).

In this context, my focus is more on women than men drug users. I have maintained this focus not because I see women as passive victims, or because I want to create a women's ghetto or define a homogenous category 'women' in opposition to 'men'. Rather, I want to understand understated, if not ignored gendering processes at work in our field. While both women and men drug users will experience the damaging effects of gender, whether as a social process or an institution, women are at a greater disadvantage because 'masculinist' (that is, male privileging) more than gender-sensitive structures and paternalistic epistemologies predominate (Ettorre, 1994). These structures and epistemologies pervade all our theories and practices, as well as determine any new developments within both classical and postmodern paradigms.

For example, we often overlook women's 'resistance' to gender and their moral critiques of society when we use deviant or medical models. These models, emerging from classical paradigms, tend to silence individuals by focusing on pathologies. More importantly, these models fail to take into account the importance of the broader social issues in which drug use is embedded (Friedman and Alicea,

2001: 3), gender being one of them. Gender-sensitive theories that analyse difference, domination and subversion as ways of looking at drug users' conditions and experiences challenge these obsolete models.

Embodiment: managing flesh and inscribing politics

Social behaviour at all times manifests itself in the fleshy human form. The body is a means of expression of who we are and who we are to become. How our bodies move in societies is shaped by complex cultural and social values and practices. Furthermore the body has become a fundamental feature of taste and distinction (Turner, 1992) in which its management is an important part of physical and cultural capital (Bourdieu, 1984). The body has been crafted with dimensions and attributes which are the result of painstaking work by anatomists and clinicians and public health officials over the years (Armstrong, 2002: 16). Embodiment scholars, such as the sociologists Bryan Turner (1996) and Chris Shilling (1993), imagine the human body as politically inscribed, its physiology and morphology shaped by histories and practices of containment and control.

Within the history of sociology, Shilling (2005: 10) notes that the 'founding fathers' implicated the body in the creation of social life as a source of properties necessary for society's inception. The problem with the notion of the body as source of society was the fundamental linkage between human capabilities and social structure: wilful intent was absent. With regard to practices of containment and control, Turner (1996: 126) contends that a sociology of the body has turned out to be, crucially, a sociological study of the control of sexuality, specifically female sexuality, by men exercising patriarchal power. Over and above this history and these controlling practices, the construction of the body as an effect of endless circulation of power and knowledge (Bordo, 1993b: 21) becomes evident. This body, this fleshy, material, human body, provides the focus for regulatory techniques applied to the individual as a material person.

In our analysis of women and drug use we need to place the body at the core of political struggles (Turner, 1996: 67). Bodies need to be seen as sites where the knowledge of drugs, women's use, femininity, negative stereotypes, reproductive functions, discourses of risk, treatment regimes and affect converge and not as gender-neutral, non-finite structures. One problem is that our work needs to be done with the explicit purpose of demonstrating how notions of 'deviant' or 'sick' gendered bodies; models of individual pathologies; gendered performances and ideas about appropriate kinds and levels of treatment are culturally dependent 'embodied processes'. Thus this work is about the need for a renaissance of the body in our work and restoring 'epistemological' existence into our abandoned frames. Our work is about upholding corporeality – making the firm contention that the body exists centrally in the drug use discourse. To make this claim is to begin to understand why the drugs field is traditionally gender-insensitive and additionally, why negative stereotypes of women users have been not only needed but also perpetuated ad infinitum.

Cyborg's trumping biopower

Until recently, explanations about women offered in the drugs field have been uncritical and ahistorical. A systematic enquiry into this issue must highlight key individual and social factors which offer full accounts of the day-to-day experiences of women drug users. We need to be able to explain comprehensibly the structural roots of power, and for women the issue of power, whether cultural, social, political or economic, is most important. In contemporary theory power is a contested concept. However, with regard to embodiment theory power has a specific pivotal point: the body is the product of power relationships. Turner (1996: 63) contends that an excursion into these sorts of power issues can be considered a materialist enquiry: this material body as an object of power is produced in order to be controlled, identified and reproduced. For Turner power manifests itself through bodily disciplines or technologies of the self and regulatory regimes targeting particular bodies, as well as entire populations. Since the Enlightenment the embodied subject has been the focal point of practices and techniques of rational scientific domination. According to Foucault this body has been at the core of productive control that marks the command of discourse in modernity and the concurrent sexualization and medicalization of the body in a new power configuration, biopower (Braidotti, 1994: 58).

Modernity is the era of biopower – of constant normativity. Biopower is about the power of normativity over living organisms; the force producing and normalizing bodies to serve prevailing relations of dominance and subordination and total control over human living matter (Braidotti, 1994: 58). In this era the body has not only exploded into a network of social practices but also imploded into a fetishized and obsessive object of care and concern (Braidotti, 2002: 229). In this complex process, the body, constructed by biopower, is many-layered and situated across multiple and opposing factors. Plainly bodies are encircled by many disciplinary regimes and strategies of attention in a relentless, incessant endeavour to normalize them.

On the other hand, contemporary power may be seen to work by means of networking, communication redesigns and multiple interconnections rather than normalized heterogeneity (Braidotti, 2002: 242). Donna Haraway (1991: 155) argues that in our fast-moving technological and scientized societies, techno-bodies or cyborgs emerge as a type of political identity, resistance or antagonistic consciousness. This identity accentuates issues of race, gender, sexual and class difference within a broad remit for survival and social justice (Braidotti, 2002: 243). This is because this cyborg identity is embodied by those refused stable race, sex and/or class membership and who have proficiency in reading 'webs of power' (Haraway, 1991: 155).

If the body is not always already there to be constructed by discourses nor its existence permanently postponed behind the meaning imposed by discourse (Shilling, 2003: 70), the body can be envisaged as Haraway's cyborg – embedded and embodied, seeking for connections and expressions in a non-gendered and non-ethnocentric perspective (Braidotti, 2002: 243). In this sense, the cyborg trumps the body confronting biopower because the cyborg is not subject to biopolitics, rather it replicates politics. The cyborg is crucial to confronting the 'informatics of domination', these frightening new networks of a world system of production, reproduction and communication (Haraway, 1991: 161–3). The cyborg is a kind of disassembled and reassembled postmodern collective and personal self – a self which, Haraway argues, feminists must code.

Whether or not one embraces Haraway's cyborg, her ideas are instructive. They teach us that women's position is deeply related to their assimilation or manipulation in this global system. Thus for feminists, that bodies really do matter in this assimilation or manipulation is about recognizing that beliefs in, discourses about and tools of modern technologies impose and embody novel social relations for women on a global scale. Most importantly for us the drug field cannot escape this type of coding, that is to say, technologies and scientific discourses about drugs and drug use can be tools for imposed, compulsory meanings and continued exploitation on the basis of race, gender and class. While drug users will be pressed into constant normativity, those with the ability to read 'webs of power' may champion their own survival and social justice and exhibit forms of 'resistance consciousness'.

The need for feminist embodiment theories on drugs

In wanting to revision women and drugs, I place gender, embodiment and power as concepts which are central to developing feminist embodiment theories on drugs. Three useful embodiment theorists, Bryan Turner (1992, 1996), Rosi Braidotti (1994, 2002) and Arthur Frank (1991, 1995, 2004), offer theoretical perspectives which link gender, embodiment and power.

Before a brief exploration of the work of these authors, it is important to point out that feminist embodiment theories provide an essential corrective to the masculinist character of much of the new body theory because we take difference, domination and subversion as starting points for understanding the conditions and experiences of embodiment in contemporary culture (Davis, 1997: 14). Kathy Davis discusses two problems that stand in the way of developing feminist embodiment theories. Firstly, there is a problem relating to grounding theories of the body in the concrete embodied experiences and practices of individual women. Davis (1997: 14) suggests that feminist theorists must capture an understanding of what embodiment means to an individual on a day-to-day basis. For her this depends upon being able to sort out how sexual, racial and other differences intersect and give meaning to one's interactions with one's body and through one's body with the world around them. Secondly there is the issue of the reflexivity of theorizing the body which involves deconstructing the body as bedrock of sexual difference, while also validating difference in order to do justice to individuals' experiences. I endeavour to address both of these problems in this context.

With regard to the first problem that Kathy Davis mentions, my embodiment theories around revisioning women and drugs take power into account. These theories are grounded in the assumption that drug use is a deeply, embodied, gendered and, for some women, racialized experience – an experience which is culturally coded and shaped. With regard to the second problem, reflexivity of theorizing the body comes into view when the tensions and contradictions between the classical and postmodernist paradigms emerge. These tensions can be used as a resource for more ruminations and explorations. For example, drug-using women's subjectivities constituted by their embodied experiences and intersections with 'difference' are constructed by a variety of constraining and conflicting expert and lay discourses, capable of being resisted, as we shall see as this book progresses. A reflexive theorizing of the female drug-using body includes a theory of the strains which a transgressive body stirs up.

As we consider feminist theories of embodiment, let us look briefly at three thinkers who link gender, embodiment and power in their work. Bryan Turner stands alone as one of the early male sociologist embodiment theorists who took women and gender seriously (see especially Turner, 1986: 82–110). In his work, Turner (1992: 35) contends that the absence of the body from social theory poses major problems for the formulation of a sociological perspective on the human agent (MAN) (*sic*), agency and human embodiment. Turner (1992: 35) contends further that if sociology is the study of action, we require a social theory of the body because human agency and interaction involve far more than knowledgeability, intentionality and consciousness. For Turner, the body is brought into culture as a potentially managed material entity in the process of ageing and a field for gender differentiation. While the body appears simultaneously as a constraint and a potential, the tensions between culture and 'natural' facts (for example, bodily needs and desires) are experienced differently according to gender (Turner, 1991: 4). Furthermore, as a result of fundamental structures of gender stratification, the political status of the human body emerges (Turner, 1991: 20) – a status bestowed more readily on white, male bodies.

In his work on chronic illness Arthur Frank (1995) argues that we must ensure that the stories we tell reflect the lives of the people we study. For him this type of behaviour is our ethical work. He contends that there is a need for an ethics of the body shaping a sociology of the body. Bodies need to be in relationship to others, especially those that are viewed as wounded bodies. Frank envisages a 'communicative body' which is the ethical ideal for wounded bodies, speaking in narratives and wanting to communicate to others by speaking as well as listening. In his view wounded women's bodies that have been silenced must break their silence, turn silence into action and become communicating 'communicative' bodies – bodies who are not afraid to share their suffering with others who respond with compassion or empathy. For Frank the epitome of the communicative body was Audre Lourde, the Black American feminist who courageously confronted her sick, suffering body by speaking and writing of her cancer publicly.

Within a materialist theory of becoming, Rosi Braidotti (2002) demonstrates that there exists a dialectical relationship between gendered bodies and the deployment of discourses generating oppressive ideas on the body. For Braidotti the material embodied subject is fragmented in these discourses, particularly the biomedical one. On the one hand, there is a shift from a metaphysical unity of the subject postulated on a careful balance of dualistic oppositions. On the other hand, there is a shift towards a multiplicity of discourses taking the embodied subject as their target (Braidotti, 1994: 46). As a result of these shifts, the female body becomes disjointed and exposed, given that complex gendered and oppressive processes are rife as dominant discourses are organized.

While absence, ethics and becoming are the key themes which emerge from Turner, Frank and Braidotti's work, respectively, Braidotti comes nearest to framing her ideas within a feminist perspective on the embodied subject. That the embodied subject has become fragmented or 'broken', as it has developed into the target of a variety of discourses and been subjected to intense scrutiny by their powerful scopic drive, is a major problem which Braidotti exposes. What is key here is that feminist embodiment theorists need to contextualize and recognize the gendered circumstances and experiences of embodiment vis-à-vis living bodies. Thus, with regard to drug use we should envisage the gendered drug-using body as the end product of a whole system of cultural relations, power, knowledge and difference. Unearthing the sorts of difficulties and tensions which this gendered drug-using body evokes is in order. One major cultural effect stirred up by this drug-using body is that it is is judged to be behaviourally abnormal or socially troublesome and, as I mentioned in a previous context, socially and culturally disabled.

Charting drug use as embodied deviance

Indispensable to our cultural and social identity, the body is the instrument for self-articulation for who we are and who we will grow to become. It is the vehicle for us to construct complex lifestyles in our consumer cultures. But scientists, policy-makers, law-makers and physicians have been averse to dealing with this material body and the notion that the body is a machine predominates. Body ideals, especially for women, are formed by ideas from history, science, medicine and consumer interests (Urla and Swedlund, 1995). Furthermore we often assess bodies according to what has been called 'benchmark man' (Brook, 1999).

In our field the vernacular of drug use relies on an individualistic, mechanistic view of a gendered body. This view goes hand in hand with the notion of embodied deviance (Urla and Terry, 1995: 2), defined as the scientific and lay claim that bodies of individuals classified as deviant are marked in some recognizable way. Here the contention is that, regardless of how deviant social behaviour is defined, it always manifests itself in the substance of the 'deviant's' body. Simply, individuals who deviate from the ideal are not only deemed to be socially and morally inferior but also their social and moral trouble-making is embodied. I want to extend these ideas into our field and link them with the earlier discussions in this chapter on gender, embodiment and power.

As a form of 'embodied deviance', drug use 'marks' bodies of individuals and determines their low social status and lack of moral agency. A drug-using body becomes a vehicle, medium or instrument for solving a variety of difficulties and problems that all bodies must face. But these difficulties and problems become exaggerated because of drug use. All bodies, whether individual bodies or groups of bodies, are involved in societal tasks that can cause internally or externally directed problems in time and space (Turner, 1996). These problems have been referred to as the four Rs (Scott and Morgan, 1993: 3): restraint, reproduction, representation and regulation. More specifically, bodies are involved in the 'internal' tasks of self-control (How do I learn to restrain or control my bodily functions such as

sexual desire, excretion, eating?) and reproduction (How will I reproduce?) and the 'external' bodily tasks of representing an acceptable
self-image (How do I present myself in an acceptable way to society?)
and regulation (How will I regulate my external behaviour?)

Restraint as a body task

In dealing with the task of self-control, an individual body asks,
'How do I learn to control my bodily functions and inner needs such
as sexual desire, excretion, eating, etc?' While the bodies of drug
users carry out this task of self-control, they have an additional task
that separates them from 'normal' bodies – obtaining their drugs,
ensuring these drugs somehow get into their bodies, avoiding risks
and managing their use. For many users, managing their use may
lead to high-risk behaviours and unstable lifestyles (Archibald, et al.,
1998). Nevertheless drug management is determined by cost, availability and source of supply, as well as different levels of bodily desires,
social exclusion and cultural engagement with a variety of drugs (see,
for example, Ditton and Hammersley, 1996; Jacobs and Miller, 1998;
Measham, Aldridge and Parker, 2001; Hammersley, Khan and Ditton,
2002). To manage one's drug use is a deeply embodied experience.
Ask any problem drinker who has the shakes, a heroin addict in
withdrawal or a body-builder whose 'ethnopharmacological knowledge' is lacking (Monaghan, 2001). This body problem of self-control
which all 'normal' bodies experience becomes for the drug user
constructed as an overwhelming, ongoing problem (Brownstein,
1995).

Most 'normal' bodies are able to resolve self-control within the
limits of 'conventional' society, as their bodies are shaped by societal
norms. As 'normal' bodies move through society, they control their
desires, passions and needs. But it is believed that drug-using bodies
are unable to do the same because their drug use is defined as 'loss
of control' (Room, 1985). This loss of control or embodied deviance
is seen to reside in their bodies as implied in the notion of 'excessive
appetites' (Orford, 2000). While society views users' need for drugs as
loss of control, compliance within the context of complex gendering
processes marks both female and male bodies in drug-using cultures.
For example, as they risk drug taking, male users comply with what
Collison (1996) calls hegemonic masculinity. Female users' risky drug

taking may be enacting norms of feminine conformity – to be sexually appealing, to relax or to deaden the pain of abusive relationships (Broom, 1994) and embody femininity in the 'nocturnal genderscape' (Henderson, 1997: 96) of clubland. While resistance and rebellion may mark male more than female bodies, the bodies of females can be seen as pleasure-seeking and hedonistic (Henderson, 1997, 1999; Measham, Aldridge and Parker, 2001; Measham, 2002), as well as a fundamental part of the gendered drug culture of resistance and self-control.

Reproduction as a body task

Bodies confront the task of reproduction. As bodies reproduce themselves, society sets conditions for this reproduction (Rothman, 1989: 39). We all have to decide in which way we will or will not reproduce. For drug users, reproduction becomes a complicated body issue because drug use is not seen as conducive to making babies or even supportive of family life (Fortney, 1990). Making a decision to reproduce is overlaid with ideologies concerning what sorts of bodies should reproduce. Drug-using bodies do not fall within those seen as highly reproductive for a variety of moral and medical reasons (Curet and Hsi, 2002).

In carrying out this bodily task of reproduction, more female than male users are at a disadvantage because, similar to 'normal' non-drug-using women (Purdy, 1996), they are viewed as fetal containers. Additionally, unlike 'normal' non-drug-using women, pregnant drug users' bodies are viewed as lethal fetal containers. While pregnant heroin users may approach their pregnancies with less anxiety than pregnant women who smoke crack, the medical construction of their bodies as toxic to their fetuses applies to all drug-using female bodies (Murphy and Rosenbaum, 1999).

Furthermore the issues of stigma and discrimination, as well as race, gender, and socioeconomic status, must be addressed if these pregnant bodies who use drugs or are at risk of HIV infection are to be helped (Abercrombie and Booth, 1997). In this context, Murphy and Rosenbaum (1999) in their excellent book *Pregnant women on drugs: combating stereotypes and stigmas*, demonstrate how pregnant drug users are the focus of social-policy concerns and the targets of treatment regimes and the law. Whether their babies are taken from them after birth or they are told to have an abortion, be sterilized, and so on, these bodies are viewed as not fit to reproduce. This is a gendered as well as an ethical issue. Simply our bodies are ourselves. Women, whether we are drug users or not, have a basic human right to reproduce – full stop!

Representation as a body task

A body must deal with its self-image by presenting oneself in an itself acceptable way in society. 'I must dress myself in culturally accepted ways.' Social success usually depends upon one's ability to manage the self by the adoption of appropriate interpersonal skills and the presentation of an acceptable image (Turner, 1996: 124). On the one hand, for the 'normal' body, this task is pretty straightforward and one follows the styles and consumer requirements of one's culture. On the other hand, while a drug user may appear, at times, as respectable (that is, is clean, courteous, well-behaved, and so on), risky consumption of risky products shape the body in physically recognizable ways. Think of the emaciated stereotype of the heroin or amphetamine user, the beer gut of the beer drinker, the wrinkled eyes of the smoker or the inflated muscles of the steroid-using body builder (Bunton and Burrows, 1995). For drug users dealing with one's self-image by representing oneself to society becomes a problem.

Presentation of self in a good enough way depends upon the drugs one uses, how and where they are administered, and the effects they have on one's body, as well as one's race, sex and class. Popular accounts of users' risk of contracting HIV or Hepatitis C convert most young users (Patton, 1995) and those selling sex (Pearce, 1999) into deviant bodies in danger of harm. Plumridge and Chetwynd (1999) note that risk is key to social interaction in narratives of users. Heroic individualism or sensual hedonism embodied men's stories, and escapes from pain or psychological drives (that is, having addictive personalities) embodied women's. These stories were shaped by an embodied sense of personal and social agency that was gendered. Agency was very present for male bodies, shaped by heroic or hedonistic identities, while it was largely lacking for females whose drug use was seen as being at the mercy of personalized, inner drives. Nevertheless earlier work (Ettorre, 1992; Henderson, 1997; Measham,

2002; Hammersley, Khan and Ditton, 2002; Hammersley et al., 1999) emphasizes sensual hedonism as embodied by female drug users whose recreational use is marked by personal agency and pursuit of pleasure.

Regulation as a body task

How do bodies regulate themselves when they confront a variety of social problems related to urban life? In asking this question bodies are bound up in society's values of discipline and order, viewed as indispensable to health and well being. Bodies must regulate their external behaviours and be attentive in space to social anonymity, as well as interpersonal intimacy (Turner, 1996: 118). To maintain and nurture bodies, as well as to labour, consume and be at leisure, requires regulation and stability. Drug-using bodies appear as those bodies which have failed in regulating their external behaviours (Smart, 1984) and internal drives. They are viewed as high risk with high needs (Bean and Neimitz, 2004). Drug-using bodies themselves become a social problem in urban cultures as attempts are made to get these polluted bodies off the streets (Murji, 1999). Drug taking is seen as a threat to the integrity of urban life, while being a fundamental part of urban consumption (Collison, 1996).

While we may be aware that both female and male users have active roles when regulating their drug behaviour in bodily routines (see, for example, Measham, Aldridge and Parker, 2001: 92–116), the embodied drug routines they engage in are seen to conflict with what is 'normal' social behaviour. On the fringes of society, drug-using bodies learn to adapt their drug behaviour to their everyday lives. But 'stable' systems of inequalities, such as gender, race and class, will shape the ways in which their already 'marked' bodies do this adaptation. Guy, a young lad of 20, in the book *The user* (Macfarlane, Macfarlane and Robson, 1996: 58) reveals the subtle gendering processes in the everyday 'doing' of drugs. For him, boys or men are the 'real' users as they are getting off their faces, while timidity embodies girls' and female regulation. Guy says:

> Drugs are a boy's thing, even if the experimentation rates are similar. The people running it, dealing in it, and the people doing

the most drugs, are boys. In addition to the bonding, there's the appeal of having a business to make money out of, and there's the drama side which people get a real rush from. Girls may try one spliff, or half an E or something, which will be enough for them, while their men will be getting completely off their faces.

On the other hand, Rachel, a sixteen year old quoted in the same book, evidences perhaps a more sophisticated approach to her drug use, an approach which evidences a conscious embracing of 'embodied deviance':

> Drugs are a definite escape – from boring normality. They've also got something to do with going against society. It's another one of those little things you're going to do so that you're not like everyone else. Every new drug I take seems to show me a new side to my personality . . . (Macfarlane, Macfarlane and Robson, 1996: 5)

The body needs to be seen as the place where we organize tasks of restraint, reproduction, regulation and reproduction. As we have seen, drug-using bodies are socially and politically shaped, while, along with Turner (1996: 67), I make the claim that we need to place the body at the centre of our analyses. In making this claim I want to confirm the complexities of gender as a process and an institution and keep the notions of embodiment and power in focus.

In conclusion, in this chapter I have defined the key notions of gender, embodiment and power that I see as the building blocks for constructing feminist embodiment theories on drugs. I have also argued that there is a need for these theories and demonstrated how the notion of 'embodied deviance' can be expanded theoretically in relation to four bodily tasks. This exploration provided important insights into the workings of the gendered body culture of drug use. Academic feminists have exposed that the traditional neglect of the body reflected a masculinist social science that naturalized bodies and furthermore legitimated control of male over female bodies. This neglect affects how we see the type of provocation and resistance experienced by gendered bodies confronting drugs. As well as continuing to develop a feminist embodied approach to drugs, I will in the following chapter analyse a series of additional notions related to women drug users through the lens of embodiment. These notions provide additional conceptual armaments in our quest for feminist embodiment theories on drugs. It is my sincere desire that these excursions into theory should bear witness to the day-to-day realities of the lives of women drug users.

3
Punishing or Privileging Marginalization?

> Much of Western European history conditions us to see human differences in simplistic opposition to each other: dominant/subordinate, good/bad, up/down, superior/inferior. In a society where the good is defined in terms of profit rather than in terms of human need, there must always be some group of people who through systematized oppression can be made to feel surplus, to occupy the place of the de-humanized inferior.
>
> Audre Lorde (1984: 245–50)

Women drug users as our co-social theorists

In a similar vein to the previous chapter, I want to explore key notions which need to be re-worked and re-shaped in the development of feminist embodiment theories on drugs. My aim is to ensure that these notions and ideas reflect the knowledge, know-how and interests of women drug users, who have been traditionally marginalized in terms of both treatment and research practice in the drugs field. Given that a reconsideration of the subjects and authors of research are crucial within the postmodern paradigm, questions around who clarifies, decodes, prioritizes and has possession of research and research outputs are crucial.

Very often, we as researchers believe that we have an almost inalienable right to gather sensitive personal information, such as drug use history, family history, accommodation status, physical health, mental health status, relationship history, reproductive history, and so on, from the women drug users that we research. Often we do this uncritically without any serious analysis of how we present these data and who benefits from the research that we carry out. With regard to this sensitive issue, my personal preference has been consistently to offer a particular view: if we want to further social justice for women drug users we need to see them as our 'co-social theorists'. We need to include them very centrally when we consider new information, create knowledge and write up our research findings. Indeed, knowledge creation and production is a politically charged activity with both personal and cultural ramifications which we share with our 'co-theorists'.

With these ideas about theory creation in mind, I want in the following discussions to consider an oppositional discourse which confronts relations of dominance and subordination vis-à-vis women and drugs. I envisage this consideration as integral to the development of feminist embodiment theories on drugs. Specifically in this chapter I will continue to analyse various notions related to women drug users and look particularly at four notions: pollution, dependence, cultures of emotion and pleasure. In examining these four notions, I want to foster a view from the margins. I want to begin to 'trouble the connections between how knowledge is created, what knowledge is produced and who is entitled to engage in these processes' (Brown and Strega, 2005: 7). My assumption is that troubling these connections and bringing a marginal view into the drugs field is essential if we are to offer alternative ways of being for women drug users.

This chapter is divided into five main discussions. I begin by defining in turn each of the key notions in four related discussions. In the final part of the chapter I attempt to create the bare bones of an oppositional discourse. In that context, I will weave together these concepts and want to privilege subjugated knowledge about women and drugs in our field. I will suggest how the conditions of women drug users' lives can be transformed by re-working, resisting or embracing these notions. Throughout this chapter, women drug users, who more often than not are marginalized and encounter a punishment approach to their drug use (Young, 1994), will remain in the forefront. As I noted earlier, I consider these gendered, racialized and classed bodies as my co-social theorists and I want them to be there in spirit on each page.

Pollution: contesting a punishing view

In earlier work (Ettorre, 1992), I contended that a hierarchy of drugs exists in the drugs field which implies that strong moralizing features are embedded in the popular discourse on drugs. Here the idea that a number of drugs or addictive substances are superior, as well as more polluting both pharmacologically and culturally than other substances, is implied. Thus there are substances ranging from 'good or more socially accepted drugs' such as alcohol and tranquillisers at the top of the hierarchy, and 'bad or unacceptable ones, such as cocaine and heroin at the bottom. It has been interesting in recent years to notice how cigarettes have slid down the hierarchy, given their harmful effects (Plant, Plant and Mason, 2002). This hierarchy of drugs is linked with our cultural value system and archaic notions of pollution and purity. While both men and women drug users are affected by this hierarchy, the social delineation of public and private spaces situates women's more than men's bodies in socially weak positions if these female bodies choose to consume what are viewed as 'bad' substances.

In a classic article, Warburton (1978) defined internal pollution as the 'state when the security of the internal environment of our bodies is destroyed'. While Warburton noted that internal pollution had received scant attention in the drugs field at that time, he argued that it was easy for those with a knowledge of drugs in society to blame over-prescribing doctors; criticize the marketing strategies of the pharmaceutical and/or the alcohol industry and see the failure of governments to curb, if not control the illegal global trade in heroin. While Warburton's ideas are rather outdated now, he characterized a notion which thrives in contemporary culture. For him, the consumers of drugs were to be blamed for internally polluting their bodies which became the interior environments for contamination. More importantly for him, drug users conspired in this pollution process by insisting on taking drugs. While this moral judgement was made and drug users were seen to pollute themselves, as well as their social environments, they involved themselves in a subtle discrimination process.

If we translate Warburton's ideas on internal pollution into today's popular culture, we are able to challenge damaging views of women drug users. Drug-using women are seen as 'polluted women' and they have become the main targets in the above discrimination process. Furthermore why is it that, in comparison to men drug users, women appear more as targets of this discrimination process? In a timeless piece, Mary Douglas (1966: 113), the British anthropologist, defined pollution as 'a type of danger which is unlikely to occur except where the lines of structure (i.e. cultural boundaries) are clearly defined'. She suggests these cultural boundaries are more obviously classified for women than for men. Given this, we could argue that the consequence of transgressing these boundaries (that is, polluting their bodies through drugs, seen to be out of control, and so on) for women drug users is social exclusion on a massive scale. In a real sense, these women are seen to have polluted or soiled identities. Furthermore pollutants such as drugs are coded as dirt or symbolic matter out of place. As a result, drug-using women can be seen to engage in a state of ritual impurity which is dangerous to themselves or others and which inheres in certain life events and conditions (that is, reproduction, family life, and so on) (Jewkes and Wood, 1999).

We all know or should be aware at least of the low, irreversible status of the female drug user. While women have the disagreeable social function of carriers of difficult emotions, historically they have been punished when these emotions were overstated or they appeared too troublesome (Chesler, 1994). Additionally, in the private/female sphere of domestic life, women, particularly mothers, are the primary emotional copers – a reality which has a long-term effect on women's psychic lives (Ernst and Goodison, 1997). These social functions and resultant cultural practices have particular consequences for women drug users. Regardless of when, where, how and why women take drugs, they are viewed as having polluted their identities and their bodies as women. In turn, they have contaminated the private space of family life and the public space of community or public hygiene.

Thus, in a popular sense, women drug users' bodies are perceived as being eminently polluted. Additionally, if a woman is pregnant, as are some women drug users, she represents a body which is 'doubly polluted'. She is doubly polluted because she consumes illegal drugs contaminating her body. In turn, these drugs are seen to have further contaminated her fetus. Unlike non-drug-using women's bodies, pregnant drug users' bodies are viewed as less than responsible vessels. These bodies are 'endangerers', if not potential murderers. This is particularly true if something drastic goes wrong and a fetus does not survive until birth. Indeed, these women are envisaged as 'conduits of harm', increasingly blamed and held responsible for damage to their children whom they have placed in harm's way even before birth (Campbell, 1999: 898)

In this context, Carter (2002) contends that women drug users bear three 'stigmata': – 'they are immoral, sexually indiscrete and inadequate care givers'. These stigmata become even more punitive when women use drugs during pregnancy. Here researchers (Paone and Alperen, 1998) have shown that women who use illicit drugs, particularly those who use them while pregnant, have traditionally been pigeonholed as immoral and unfit for parenting. These authors note that particularly in the United States there has been an unprecedented backlash against pregnant drug users, as well as a campaign to punish them through civil and criminal action. This is all done in a manner which is plagued with racial and gender bias.

Here, while the female body is the epitome of women's reproductive nature, drug use is seen as an assault on women's bodies. A drug-using woman becomes the cultural representation of a contemporary woman who does not care enough about her body. Furthermore she can be seen to have 'womb dirtiness' and be involved in a complex, 'ethno-pathological process', the representation of a 'general idiom' through which disease is expressed (Jewkes and Wood, 1999). Indeed, as a drug user she is viewed as a ritually diseased, marginalized citizen and an eminently polluted female body.

Dependence: swinging both ways

A very basic theme of feminist thinking is that women more than men are socialized into dependency and, as Carol Gilligan (1987: 57) has noted, a 'woman's place is in a man's life cycle'. This idea of women's dependency must be understood in cultural, economic, social and political contexts as multi-pervasive. In related contexts (Ettorre, 1989a, 1989b, 1992), I detailed the tandem definitions of 'dependency' and discussed with special reference to the drugs field the delicate and complex implications of these dual meanings for women. To aid an understanding of these subtleties I will explain briefly the ideas I presented in those previous, related contexts.

Concisely, the etymological roots of the English word 'dependency' are the Latin words 'de' and 'pendere', meaning 'to hang down from'. However, there are two meanings of dependence in the English language: 'habit'/'addiction' or 'a subordinate thing'. For women, the former meaning (habit or addiction) is what I have referred to as the unacceptable side of dependency, while the latter meaning (of the 'subordinate thing' kind) is the acceptable side of dependency, as well as a cultural norm for most, if not all women. For example, dependency (of the addiction kind) is socially 'unacceptable' when it gets in the way of a woman's social functioning, for instance as grandmother, aunt, mother, daughter, cousin, worker, carer, driver, sportsperson, and so on, while dependency (of the 'subordinate thing' kind) is seen to be valued or 'culturally good enough' when it involves being dependent on a man, men, male sexuality, male protection, male bosses or masculinist structures. For any woman, the cultural expectation that she will conduct herself in traditional, that is, dependent, ways is clear.

Nevertheless an incongruity exists between the cultural expectation that women be dependent and the need for all women to be in charge of their lives. For example, women, by being dependent on male kinship structures, such as the family, can be viewed as being constrained, if not controlled by men (whether consciously or not) (Yanagisako and Collier, 2004). While being constrained structures her life, she is still perceived as being in control. In this context a woman drug user may consciously choose to use an addictive substance in order to cope with or control an oppressive, controlling situation such as her family life, an intimate relationship or even to be better mothers (Baker and Carson, 1999: 360). Regardless of how she sees herself, she is viewed as 'a woman out of control' and not a 'normal' woman. The basic cultural message for a woman is that, at all times, she should be in control of herself, mindful of her partner, her children, her home responsibilities and her work. If she feels strung out, stressed or unable to cope, she should avoid addictive substances.

On a more wide-ranging level, this issue of dependency becomes more multifaceted when we consider that women's dependent status is contingent upon their being at the same time depended upon by others. For women deeply involved in the social organization of caring, giving care and helping others is a fundamental part of being a dependant. Her caring body is viewed not only as a dependent body but also a dependable body – a resource. In some ways this illustrates the cultural complexities of dependency for women. Perhaps, in this light, we are able to see that in relation to women drug users the word 'dependency' has various hues of meaning and cultural representations in both public and private spaces, as well as with regard to female embodiment. In this context, one author (Copeland, 1998: 331) demonstrates that women drug users' socialization into dependency relationships with men is all about attempts to attain happiness or at least an embodied need to succumb to intense social pressures concerning what is expected of them as women.

When we consider this issue of dependency in relation to Black, ethnic minority and indigenous women, our focus must shift to include a perspective on terror vis-à-vis dependency. Here we need to understand the capacity of White supremacy (hooks, 1996) to inspire terror amongst those who are not White, as well as the overriding power of colonialist ways of thinking to confuse dependency with the right to dominate. Simply, in Black, ethnic minority and indigenous contexts we must recognize how a clear picture of women, drugs and dependency is obscured by the cultural constraints and undeniable destructiveness of White racism. If racialized cultures, including family forms, social relationships, and so on, serve as a model of abnormality against which nationalism or whiteness is constructed (White, 2001: 122), and furthermore drug use serves as a model of disease against which health is measured, both kinds of dependency are terrorizing experiences for Black, ethnic minority and indigenous women (and some men). It is important that this is recognized and understood by social theorists in the drugs field.

Cultures of emotions

The traditional neglect of the body in the social sciences reflects masculinist and colonialist preconceptions that naturalize bodies, while legitimating male control over female bodies, as well as White governance over Black bodies. In this context, we saw in the previous chapter how drug use as a form of 'embodied deviance' shapes bodies of individuals and determines their low social status and lack of moral agency. We also saw how all bodies are implicated in societal tasks that can cause trouble and how the drug-using body needs to be seen as the place where we organize tasks of restraint, representation, regulation and reproduction.

All these ideas need to be contextualized further with an awareness of risk. Simply, gendered, drug-using bodies are culturally and politically shaped by disciplinary practices within the context of an economy of difference, as well as an economy of risk. With regard to the bodies of women drug users, these practices shape women's bodies as 'damaged bodies'. I use the term 'damaged bodies' to suggest that White, male, Eurocentric or Western ways of thinking have been based on separating ourselves from our bodies as cultural and moral actors. Furthermore, we – especially women – have become disembodied in our ways of theorizing (Braidotti, 1994). Morality is highly mediated by gender and it has been traditionally based on the exclusion of female bodies from extensive moral agency. Consequently, in moral terms women experience a fragmented morality of the body. Women's bodies are not whole; they have become 'broken', damaged and subjugated.

As Donna Haraway (1991: 199) notes, 'When female "sex" has been so thoroughly re-theorized and re-visualised that it emerges as practically indistinguishable from "mind" something basic has happened to the category of biology'. Thus the biological politics of the body, particularly the female body, have been altered as the body has become the agent through which we form partial perspectives about our affective or emotional lives. There is a discernible need to make sentient bodies visible within the politics of drug use. Until this is done we will have an incomplete understanding of how the affective politics of drug use sustains women's subordination through love, trust and intimacy (MacRae and Aalto, 2000) within the context of risky and chaotic, heteronormative relationships and engagement in a whole series of cultural and institutionalized practices.

In our field we need to document the types of regulation, restraint, provocation and resistance experienced by gendered, racialized, classed bodies confronting drugs. The cultural outrage levelled against women drug users is one more moral deployment in the stigmatization and hatred of women's drug-using bodies. To consume drugs is to open oneself up to risk (Collison, 1996). However, this type of cultural outrage can also be an occasion for female bodies to privilege their performativities of disgust (that is, drug use) (Ahmed, 2004); to access their own raw materials of emotion and awarenesses of risk; to consume actively but carefully and to create a particular lifestyle that has traditionally remained undeveloped and repressed in drug-using environments.

However, in looking at the affective dimensions of risk or, more simply, drug-using women's 'cultures of emotions', we see permeable boundaries existing between precarious emotions and past, present and future risks in their drug-using worlds. (See Chapter 8 for a more detailed discussion on emotions and drug use.) For these women embodied emotions can be an important resource which challenges the governing mentalities (Campbell, 2000) and disciplinary framework of current drug policies. Whether or not consumption of drugs produces desire without pleasure (Caan, 2002: 181), women are able to use drugs for pleasure, as we shall see in the following discussion. Drug-using women do not necessarily need to view their actions as deviant. Indeed, embodied emotions can be a form of pleasure, as evidenced in recent research (Hinchliff, 2001) which found that ecstasy was used as a form of independent pleasure by women drug users. On an affective level, this idea appears to contradict traditional research findings within the classical paradigm. This is mainly because emotional or affective dimensions of women drug users' lives have been subverted or concealed along with the knowledge that drug use can be born out of a need to extinguish unrelenting emotional pain, especially for racialized women (R. Davis, 1997). Do we see these ideas as scandalous or equally as an important issue that is productive of social and cultural theory? We need to consider all sorts of possibilities for women drug users, especially if we want to embrace an embodiment approach.

Pleasure: a crucial notion or not?

Regardless of the perceived wisdom in the drugs field, drug use involves pleasure. In earlier work (Ettorre, 1992) I asked the question whether or not the issue of substance use and pleasure was relevant for women. While my answer was 'yes' in that prior context, I wanted to be clear that I was not advocating drug use. I was merely proposing that it is important in our work to look at the pleasurable effects of drugs side by side the tenderness which its painful consequences can evoke. Thus we need to recognize that, regardless of any changes within our drug cultures, women drug users' negotiation of femininity, risk and pleasure in relation to their sexualities and drug use will continually be problematic (Hutton, 2004). While my own interest in drug use and pleasure began in the early 1990s (see Ettorre, 1992), it has taken a long time for other researchers to develop a similar interest and in this light I contend that their lack of interest in pleasure is due to a variety of reasons.

First, drug use is perceived generally by non-users and users alike as too much of a stigmatized activity to be considered pleasurable and they have ignored exploring this notion. To bring pleasure into this activity is viewed as not acceptable, confusing or intolerable. Nevertheless drugs researchers do recognize how drug use is an important cultural issue with moral meanings attached. They are aware that drug use indicates a form of 'disreputable pleasure' (O'Malley and Vlaverde, 2004) and this fact is beginning to be acknowledged.

Secondly, often pleasure is linked with desire and this link conjures up notions of sexuality, sexual intercourse or erotic yearnings. While the experience of ecstasy users in popular culture tends to be sexualized, sexual pleasure for heroin users is bounded by moralistic notions which sanction, if not prohibit, sexual intercourse or penetration with or without condoms. It is almost as if these heroin users forfeit their right to pleasurable sex and if they have sex it should be experienced in its most ignoble form as 'exchange for something'. In this sense, drug users are seen to embody bad sex, desperate attempts at human intimacy or base human genital materiality. When applied specifically to female drug-using bodies, these moralistic notions become even more pejorative. While female bodies are perceived to lack full moral agency, these bodies more than men's have been shaped as guardians of morals. On the other hand, Mulia's (2000: 757) work has shown that women drug users are able to experience the pleasures of sex, even under conditions of pressing material needs. While women drug users' sexual relations can contain elements of 'exchange for something', these relationships may also include rudiments of friendship, caring and emotional attachment.

Thirdly, notions of pleasure are often linked with what embodied subjects, drug-using or not, do in their leisure time, and looking at what drug users do in their leisure time has not been a research priority (Parker, Aldridge and Measham, 1998; Parker, Measham and

Aldridge, 1995). Indeed, if consumption of leisure were acknowledged and indeed accepted, it would bring the theorists closer to a more normalized view of drug use (Parker, 2005). Using a European typology, Jason Ditton and Martin Hammersley (1996) speak of 'leisure type' cocaine users as opposed to 'cocainist types', who centre their lives around cocaine. In research and treatment terms, the 'cocainist types' were traditionally of most interest and curiosity, while 'leisure types' appeared to fall by the wayside. If leisure is associated with recreational drug use, it may be transformed into 'illegal leisure', creating a visible tension between normalized and deviant bodies, as implied above (Parker, Aldridge, and Measham, 1998). And it appears that this has to be avoided at all costs. The drugs field cannot accommodate the idea that deviant drug-using bodies can be similar to non-drug-using ones, or that leisure can be a factor in one's use. Furthermore, in drug treatment contexts leisure is not only viewed as gendered but racialized (Walton, Blow and Booth, 2001), making the notion of pleasure a more complicated, if not shunned issue in White, male, hegemonic clinical settings.

There are probably more reasons than those offered above for drug researchers' lack of exploration of the links between pleasure and drugs. However, regardless of the resistance to the notion of pleasure in our drugs field, in recent years researchers have started to explore this link. What I find interesting in these explorations is that the majority of researchers are more often than not focusing on female rather than male bodies in developing their notions of pleasure and drug use. This evidences a rather obvious slide to naturalizing bodies. Simply, the belief is perpetuated that in comparison to male drug-using bodies, female bodies are shaped more as embodying pleasure or at least the potential for pleasure. This is regardless of the fact that a hegemonic principle of pleasure as duty is imposed on both genders (Lury, 1996), while they attempt a delicate balance between creativity and constraint in their everyday, localized routines and practices of consumption (Mackay, 1997: 10). I would contend that, within drug consumption cultures, contemporary women appear perhaps as more receptive to transforming their views of traditional femininity. More importantly, in comparison to men, women's receptivity may activate an increased sense of agency, if not pleasure.

For example, in looking at the club scene in the North of England, Fiona Hutton (2004: 236) speaks of a 'positive femininity' where pleasure is found by women in the friendly social atmosphere of underground club spaces and spending time with friends. While women's drug use is a source of risk, it is also a source of pleasure and, more importantly, a means by which women actively challenge traditional modes of femininity. These clubbing female bodies take pleasure by avoiding risk. In a related context, earlier work by Sheila Henderson (1993) demonstrates how women 'feminize' their drug use by combining it with activities such as fashion seeking, clothes consumption, music and dance into a cultural space demarcated by pleasure and 'fun'. How women drug users embody a type of sensual hedonism – their recreational use marked by personal agency and pursuit of pleasure (Henderson, 1996) – becomes clear. In a similar vein, Sharron Hinchcliff's (2001) study, mentioned earlier, exposes how pleasure is central to women's use of ecstasy and that use of drugs for enjoyment is a taken for granted reality. Looking at women users in the criminal justice system, Emma Wincup (2000) found that women's drug use is an active strategy to achieve personal and social satisfaction, to cope with life's stresses and problems and to exert some control over their lives. In her view, similar to 'all' women, drug-using women have overburdened bodies which manage pain, while at the same time seeking pleasure.

Pleasure comes through in the work of Geoffrey Hunt, Karen Joe-Laidler and Kirsty Evans (2002: 393) on San Francisco gang girls who use drugs to get high asserting their right to use drugs, party, experiment and basically take pleasure for themselves. In the Canadian context, Patricia Erikson, Jennifer Butters, Patti McGillicuddy and Ase Hallgren's (2000: 773) work is illuminating. These researchers note that, regardless of the various reasons why women initiate crack use, these women share an enthusiasm for its acute embodied effects and are happy to talk about what they like most about the drug. While embodied pleasure is clearly experienced, it is also shaped in their accounts by an embodied ambivalence or a material appreciation of its 'down side'. This theme of embodied ambivalence or the ambiguities of pleasure emerges in Fiona Measham's (2002: 360) work in which women not only consciously consume drugs for pleasure but also find, following consumption, that issues of guilt, risk and neglect plague them in their attempts to embody traditional femininity.

While pleasure in the treatment world appears to be a scarce commodity, work on identity transformation by women in drug treatment is able to expose some interesting results linked to pleasure (Baker, 2000). The process of providing a narrative of their drug addiction is the mechanism by which women in treatment are able to achieve recovery. Included in their narratives are realizations about their addictions, emotional well-being and parenting roles. By making discoveries about themselves in a supportive environment women are able to transform their identities: they achieve greater self-esteem, overall happiness and pleasure for themselves (Baker, 2000). Wherever women's drug-using bodies are placed in treatment clubs, injecting rooms, on the streets, and so on and whatever drugs they consume, these bodies need to be perceived as flexible (Martin, 1994) and responsive to changing environments and increased performance of femininities (Blum and Stracuzzi, 2004: 273). On the one hand, prescribed drug use by women in the form of Prozac may be seen to reinforce gender boundaries. On the other hand, the consuming, affective female body of the illegal drug user creates space for an imaginative form of femininity: illegal pleasures may become escapes from powerlessness and domination in everyday life and a type of consumption of desire (Ettorre, forthcoming). Additionally, drug consumption such as smoking, albeit legal, can be experienced as an embodied form of female resistance to traditional femininity (Wearing, Wearing and Kelly, 1994).

Here we need to be cautious in any interpretations of pleasure and women's drug use. This is not only because, as we have seen, the flip side is pain, risk and danger, but also because an anti-oppressive methodology (Moosa-Mitha, 2005; hooks, 1995) reveals links between pleasure and terror for Black, ethnic minority and indigenous women. Plainly, drugs such as crack cocaine can be gendered, but these can also be racialized (Irwin, 1995). Drugs do not escape what Celia Lury (1996: 156–61) refers to as 'commodity racism'. If Whiteness is experienced by racially marginalized groups as a position of privilege in society, White privilege as well as Black marginality can easily be translated to drug-using cultures. This may create a sense of terror and dread for these racialized, gendered drug-using bodies. Perhaps here we can sense how the experience of drug use may create not only pleasure but also terror for Black, ethnic minority and indigenous women users.

I continue to be interested in why and how women experience their drug use as pleasurable. In the past, my starting point was to ask, 'What pleases women?' and in finding an answer to that question, I contended that we need to preserve what I called a view from below (Ettorre, 1992). Today I extend my earlier analysis by paying more attention to those on the margins – both those who are 'below' and those in marginalized spaces. Along with others (Moosa-Mitha, 2005: 63), I want to envisage the sorts of transformations that would occur if difference was treated as the basis rather than the site of exclusion for membership in society. If this type of transformation were to happen now, pleasure for women drug users would be visible because society would recognize these women's needs, their integrity, their human potential and, most importantly, their embodied difference.

Women, drugs and difference through the lens of feminist embodiment

In the concluding part of this chapter, I continue to weave a feminist embodiment perspective on women and drugs. Already in the previous chapter I demonstrated the need for these perspectives and theories. As we have seen, the notions of pollution, dependence and the affective dimensions of risk and pleasure work together to construct powerful images of women drug users in society. These notions allow for a level of struggle, inconsistency and instability in shaping female embodiment for women drug users. Here I want to begin my weaving by making connections with three feminist strategies which should be useful to us as researchers working in this area. These strategies represent 'the bare bones' of a practical response to ensuring a feminist embodiment perspective. They include: (i) upholding an ethics of understanding, (ii) envisaging women drug users' involvement in what Anderson (2005) calls 'core activities' as embodied activities (Ettorre, forthcoming) and (iii) making pleasure visible in the drugs field.

Upholding an ethics of understanding

While the body in a postmodern paradigm is viewed as a site of intersection between power, the corporeal flesh and the individual as subject to and of truths, we must not overlook the gendering of truths in this power/knowledge nexus (Shildrick, 1997). When we weave these embodiment ideas together with ideas in the drugs world, we must continue to be vigilant in noticing how drug-using bodies may stand for something fundamentally male or fundamentally female and how this can be taken as a biological and moral given. Here we are able to sense how naturalizing tends to raise its ugly head.

It is important that within the postmodern paradigm a feminist embodiment perspective on drug use offers a critical approach incorporating a vision of culture which upholds the importance of gender as a key theoretical issue, as well as an embodied and embedded social practice. Here a feminist embodiment perspective needs an ethics of understanding. This sort of understanding requires an anti-oppressive methodology which preserves a vision of gender as both a social process and a cultural institution and makes a political onslaught on the obvious and often violent workings of class and race. By crafting an ethics of understanding we create an 'ethical moment' (Shildrick, 1997: 216). In this ethical moment we flush out modernist notions of static, unchanging bodies, as well as complete, fulfilled identities marked by these kinds of stagnant bodies. In this moment we also create feminist space. Our ethics of understanding encompasses a knowledge of drug use which allows an awareness of embodied, gendered, racialized selves to emerge. On a very practical level this means we learn to appreciate and understand the ways in which different types of women drug users think through their deviant bodies.

Envisaging women drug users' 'core activities' as embodied

We saw how a drug-using woman becomes the cultural representation of a contemporary woman who does not care enough about her body. We also saw how she appears as a polluted body, particularly if she becomes pregnant. Linked with the notion of dependence, her 'polluted' caring body is viewed not only as a dependent body but also as a body which should be dependable vis-à-vis her significant others. Here it is interesting to note, with special reference to the sorts of 'core activities' (Anderson, 2005) (for example, control of the household; their purchasing 'power'; subsidizing men's use and engaging in dealing) that women drug users are involved in, how these activities can be conceptualized as resources or 'embodied' caring work (Ettorre, forthcoming). (These 'core activities' will be discussed in more detail in the following chapter.) Additionally, in focusing on these core activities as embodied resources, we are able to move beyond traditional assumptions surrounding women's contributions to drug cultures.

That drug-using bodies can be seen as the end-product of a whole system of power relations (Armstrong, 1987: 66) is significant but perhaps obvious. Nevertheless embedded within these social and cultural processes are boundaries between normal and deviant bodies. The notion of 'core activities' blurs these boundaries for women drug users. The cultural, social and punishing components of the drug-misuse orthodoxy shape abnormal, gendered drug-using bodies as distinct from normal gendered, non-drug-using ones. In these processes a variety of disciplinary strategies attend to female drug-using bodies to construct and attempt to normalize them. But their involvement in 'core activities' challenges this orthodoxy, while exposing that these disciplinary strategies emerge from outdated social theories and cultural representations of women drug users.

Putting women's 'core activities' into perspective, as well as bringing the body into our work will allow us to challenge the drug misuse orthodoxy. In practice this means that we keep a vigilant eye on how gendered, racialized, deviant bodies are able to rise above drug use as 'an epidemic of the will' by embracing 'the pathos ridden narrative of kicking the habit' (Sedgwick, 1994: 130); recognizing their marginalization as both relational and structural and envisaging core practices or activities as embodied resources.

Making pleasure visible

If using drugs, as well as healing from drugs, brings pleasure then so be it. Nevertheless, users, treaters, researchers and theorists in the drugs field need to challenge the general fear of pleasure, as well as the reticence to explore its consequences. While privileged groups in consumer society urge a morality of pleasure as duty (Lury, 1996: 100), women drug users need to defy the cultural need to work at pleasure. As I argued in an earlier context (Ettorre, 1992), women drug users need to see the potential for effective social action in de-privatizing their pain, while making their pleasure more culturally visible. I argued in that earlier context that there existed a need to make public women's experience of 'patriarchal pain' and how women's drug use as a 'private pleasure' was borne out of this 'patriarchal pain', encountered by many women.

Today, while I would uphold the existence of 'patriarchal pain', I would shift focus from a perspective that contests difference (and possibly perpetuates dominance) to a perspective that contests all forms of oppression that are structural, relational and cultural in nature (Moosa-Mitha, 2005: 62). Yes, pleasure needs to be made more visible. But making pleasure more visible means exploring the contested regions of structural and cultural relations that relate to difference, as well as crossing those intellectual boundaries which we are often afraid to cross. This means acknowledging that in theorizing about women and drug use I recognize that I can be both oppressed as well as oppressor and that I am immune neither from strategies of resistance nor from creating privileging frameworks.

In conclusion, drug-using bodies, specifically female ones, need to be considered as deeply involved with the issues of pollution, dependence, cultures of emotion and pleasure. As drug-use theoreticians and, for some of us, as feminists, we should envisage social interactions in these areas as being culturally dependent embodied processes. Our work should be about the affirmation of gendered corporeality, making the distinct claim that the body, and specifically embodied emotions, risk, power, knowledge shaped by gender, race and class exist very centrally in discourses on women and drugs. While recognizing the need to bring the body into the drug field, I see that all sorts of activities in which we are involved as social beings are embodied activities. I would suggest that what gendered, racialized and classed drug-using bodies experience, suffer, bear, desire and consume should be the foundation stones for feminist embodiment studies in the drug field. Indeed, as we have seen, pain and suffering, as well as pleasure and human longing, should not be left out of the equation. Perhaps one thing is becoming clear: the bodies of women drug users are constantly disciplined within an overpowering, moralizing discourse on drugs. These women drug users are sexualized and medicalized as a 'bio-underclass' (Baker and Carson, 1999: 349). Their access to cultural, social, political or economic power is mediated not only by their damaged views of themselves (Dale and Emerson, 1995) and their own despair (Spittal and Schechter, 2001) but also by their lack of access to an extensive range of material, cultural and social resources needed to live a satisfying life (Kandall, 1996). Let us hope, as our co-social theorists, drug-using women will have the strength to resist oppression and move towards privileging marginality. We need to help them in this worthwhile endeavour.

4
Embodying Core Activities: Gendered Performativities

> Femininity pleases men because it makes them appear more masculine by contrast; and in truth, conferring an extra portion of unearned gender distinction on men, an unchallenged space in which to breathe freely and feel stronger, wiser, more competent is femininity's special gift. One could say that masculinity is often an effort to please women, but masculinity pleases by displays of mastery and competence while femininity pleases by suggesting that these concerns, except in small matters are beyond its intent.
>
> Susan Brownmiller (1984: 4)

Being abject, being deviant

In the discussions in the previous chapters I have focused more on women than on men. This is not because I see women as passive victims, because I want to create a separate or 'essentialist' women's space or because I define a seamless theoretical category, women, in opposition to men. No. I want to uncover the sometimes obscure gendering processes at work in our field. While both women and men drug users will experience the damaging effects of these gendering processes, women are more disadvantaged than men because 'masculinist', patriarchal and paternalistic rather than gender-sensitive configurations and epistemologies predominate (Ettorre, 1994). My contention is that these gendered and gendering epistemologies permeate all our theories and practices.

In recent years these masculinist or male-privileging epistemologies and regulatory practices have been challenged by women and other scholars in the field (see, for example, Ettorre, 2004, 1992; Measham, 2002; Evans et al., 2002; Raine, 2002; Hunt, Joe-Laidler and Evans, 2002; Hunt and Evans, 2003; Murphy and Rosenbaum, 1999; Sterk, 1999; Dunlap, Tourigny and Johnson, 2000; Dunlap, Johnson and Maher, 1997; Henderson, 1996; Anderson, 2005, 1995) with the development of feminist or at least gender-sensitive perspectives. We have begun to envisage new subjectivities for women (Measham, 2002; Hammersley et al., 2002; Ettorre, 2004) across the life course (Dunlap, Tourigny and Johnson, 2000). In particular, clinicians are becoming more aware that gender is a key component of individual identity and, more significantly, that women drug users experience the world differently from men in terms of relationships, cognitive and coping styles, value systems and decision-making processes (Curet and Hsi, 2002: 75). In this context it is important to understand how women's drug use reflects aspects of their social positioning and expresses specific aspects of their gender identity (Measham, 2002).

Most, if not all, of us know that illegal drugs have distinct social spaces in diverse cultures. Regardless of the culture, society or defined social space in which illegal drug users find themselves, women drug users are viewed as more abject than men. Here abjectness is an interesting notion. Abject refers to the realm outside culture which threatens to reduce culture to chaos; 'it is shapeless, monstrous, damp and slimy, boundless and beyond the outer limits' (Brook, 1999: 14). Being abject places those perceived as such in a liminal state. Thus, when I use the term abject here I want to emphasize that women's drug use is not only emblematic of their failure as women but also confirms the essential monstrosity of their bodies (Braidotti, 1994: 81), their abjection. Abjectness is not about affirming positive aspects of female embodiment and subjectivity. On the contrary, abject denotes negativity. Being abject for a woman drug user requires that her drug-using body is disciplined by specific rituals and rules of containment, conjuring up notions of embodied, monstrous deviance, as well as deviant activities and performances.

While the engendering of bodies is being rearranged to require the increased performance of femininities by women in contemporary culture, only legal rather than illegal drug users have access to a type of productive femininity (Blum and Stracuzzi, 2004: 272–3) which is becoming visible in popular culture. This is because in the post Fordist economy the use of legal drugs, such as the drug Prozac, is not only becoming for women the corporate equivalent of steroids but also allowing women to be worthy of an enhanced productive body (Blum and Stracuzzi, 2004: 278). Nevertheless as feminist theorists we need to negotiate new boundaries for female identities in a world where power over the body has reached an implosive peak (Braidotti, 1994: 94), especially in the drugs field. We need to ask why female users of illegal drugs have little or no access to a productive body and femininity.

In this chapter, I want to continue feminist theorizing by establishing additional theoretical links with ongoing work in the drugs field and maintain my intense focus on the female body. I will look closely and critically at Tammy Anderson's (2005) novel ideas on women drug users' 'core activities' in the illicit drug world through the lens of feminist embodiment. Thus my intention is to scrutinize in detail the effects of these core activities on women's drug-using bodies. As I mentioned in the previous chapter, I am interested in how these core activities or dimensions of women's power in the illicit drug economy can be conceptualized as 'embodied' caring work, if not valuable resources. For a number of years, problems in the lives of women drug users have remained veiled. Traditional assumptions have been that men are socially dominant and active participants in the drug-using culture and women are socially subordinate and relatively passive. In this type of disciplinary regime men occupy the hegemonic space of dominant users, while women become the targets of societal rage (Kandall, 1996: 285).

In this shifting context, Anderson (1998) has argued that seeing women as defective or subordinate stunts social policy. She argues that women appear in the drugs world in different ways from men and connections between women's pursuits in the illegal and conventional worlds need to be made. By focusing on empowerment and agency Anderson (2005) contends that women perform four core activities: (i) providing shelter, housing and other sustenance needs; (ii) purchasing goods and services; (iii) subsidizing or promoting male dependency, and (iv) dealing drugs. These are viewed as fundamental to the social and economic organization of the drug world (Anderson and Levy, 2003), and for Anderson (2005) these core activities demonstrate how women gain power in the illegal drug economy.

While these activities can aid more conventional lifestyles for women drug users 'in future', the responsibility, risk management and stability implicit in these activities can be transferred to the conventional world. For Anderson (2005: 373) a focus on these core activities not only demonstrates women's empowerment and agency but also how 'their more relational power assists males' accumulation of structural power and is fundamental to successful illicit drug world organization'.

This chapter is divided into three main discussions. First, I examine how women's core activities intersect with the gendered body culture of the drug-using world. I will attempt to link Anderson's core activities with new forms of female subjectivities and embodiment and draw these into a feminist resource framework. Drug cultures are not only gendered, body cultures but also gendered spaces where the female body emerges as a site for the commonplace acts of resistance and rebellion, as well as conformity. As suggested earlier, this polluted body becomes a metaphor for failed femininity, emotionality, sexuality and a breaking down of self-risk management (Malloch, 2004). Secondly, I will offer a critique of Anderson's views and argue why an embodiment perspective is a necessary corrective to what she offers. In the concluding part of the chapter, I contend that we should continue to use critical notions of gender, embodiment and power in bearing witness to women drug users in order for them to maintain their integrity and bodies as whole.

The assumption running throughout this chapter is that a lucid awareness of women drug users' experiences of these four core activities as embodied can be useful in exploring theoretical developments of similar activities in the drugs field. Delving into the intersection of the female body, the technologies of drug use and the performance of core activities should offer us a full understanding of the contested nature of gendered representations of drug use and help us to see women's bodies as resources.

Women's core activities through the lens of embodiment

Let us now return to Anderson's four core activities which allow women drug users to enact, manage and spatialize their influence in the drug-using world. To reiterate, these core activities are: (i) providing shelter, housing and other sustenance needs;

(ii) purchasing goods and services; (iii) subsidizing or promoting male dependency, and (iv) dealing drugs. In light of the earlier discussions, I ask the question, How does the notion of gendered embodiment intersect with these core activities? Given that we have little knowledge of how gender influences the ways in which drug users coordinate their space, time, drugs, community resources, and others – whether those others be other users, relatives, families or carers – posing answers to this question is appropriate. Furthermore, a discussion of female embodiment vis-à-vis these core activities should help to demonstrate how gender can be used as a template for gathering important knowledge on drug use. Indeed, a major thread of thinking in this book is that access to drugs, knowledge of drugs, use of drugs and help for misuse of drugs all involve hidden and sometimes not so hidden gendered processes and performativities (Butler, 1990). This latter notion centres on how bodies 'perform themselves' with regard to gender. Here performativity is all about a continuing recital of exchanges between bodies and discourses. Let us now look closely at these four core activities which, when linked with an embodiment perspective, allows us to see how drug-using bodies perform themselves with regard to gender.

The domestic body – control of the household

Anderson (2005) notes that the first dimension of women's 'power' in the illicit drug economy pertains to the housing that drug-using women provide to members of inner-city drug worlds. Linked to a woman's control of the household, this core activity points to organizing the variety of physical, intimate spaces which provides refuge, emotional labour and cultural sustenance for her significant others. How does this relate to women drug users' embodiment? For a drug-using woman, she is the domesticated, instrumental and functional body in the inner city household. While many discourses (for example, biomedical, legal, media, drugs, and so on) regulate her body and shape it as a deviant, abject or 'monstrous' one, there are various technologies of the self (for example, providing a visible space for significant others, collecting material goods for her and others' subsistence, maintaining the physical structure of the home, and so on) which are at work in her desire for drugs and may relate to a stake in conventional life (Waldorf, Reinarman and Murphy 1992: 10).

Nevertheless her domestic as well as deviant embodiment disrupts dualistic thinking.

While being 'deviant female bodies', these women are not incarcerated temporally and spatially in the restricted regime of the prison – where those in the criminal justice machinery would place her if she were visible to them (Wincup, 2000). Also, the domestic sphere or the household tends to be designated as a social space demarcated more by female than male bodies. While a hybrid 'domestic masculinity' (McDowell, 2003) may exist, a female drug user, whether or not she has a sense of domestic femininity, is most likely unable to challenge the naturalized view of her regulated body within the constructed social space of the household.

In the drugs field, domesticated drug-using bodies, whether male, female or other genders may move freely between the public and private spaces of their everyday lives. However, in order to be successful domesticated bodies, women drug users need to maintain connections between what is viewed by society as their respectable or responsible (e.g. relations with their significant others, such as partner, parent, etc.) and their disrespectful, irresponsible or shameful (e.g. drug using) embodied activities. Yet, criminal justice and medical regimes do not bestow the aura of respectability on women drug users even those who are respectable or responsible within the domestic sphere. Overall, women drug users are seen to inhabit social circumstances typified by a narrowing of life's options that decreases their ability to assume conventional roles (Mullings, Marquart and Diamond, 2001).

In the hierarchies of social values (Skeggs, 1997), women drug users remain outside the realm of the respectable and are more easily classified as dangerous, bad, risky or monstrous bodies. Thus, gaining respectability while doing drugs may become problematic for these female bodies as a sense of shame or disconnection can easily become embedded in their domestic lives (Dale and Emerson, 1995).

On the one hand, they embody dependability by attending to intimate household spaces and making provisions for partners and significant others in these delineated spaces with regulated bodily regimes. On the other hand, the frailty of the boundaries between their bodies and the conventional world is evidenced by the negative consequences which may occur if fragmentation and humiliation characterize their bodily regimes both temporally and spatially. These bodily regimes reinforce continued engagement with the illicit drug world. Domestic space and its regulated temporality may be viewed as tainted by female bodies embedded in deviant lifestyles. In normative discourses these female bodies are emblematic of recklessness, lack of responsibility and unsuccessful femininity. Regardless of their ability to embody dependability and provide opportunities for their partners to accumulate resources in domestic spaces, the power of normativity is overwhelming – they are never far from its grasp.

In this context Anderson (1995) notes that this core activity provides important forms of capital for women drug users and their dependents and in the end enables successful drug careers. But this type of 'success' is based on female bodies culturally constructed in opposition to patriarchal authority and as a challenge to the continuity of male property and power. In these contexts women embody an investment strategy in the non-conventional drug culture, while carrying out conventional female, supportive activities.

While drug use may be experienced as a corporeal or bodily style, women's domesticated bodies epitomize the dual aspects of dependency (See Ettorre, 1992, and chapter 1 of this book): others are dependent upon them and they are dependent upon drugs. In this way their bodies may be resources. But these bodies are constructed to serve prevailing gendered power relations, while they are produced outside the realm of gender respectability. In effect, dependency itself becomes a bodily style for these female bodies, as their domesticated spaces are central to the social and economic organization of drugs and related embodied activities. These female bodies are relegated to becoming strategic defences against conventional society, as well as being necessary for male drug users in terms of women's own physical capital, their domesticated bodies. As Maria Esther Epele (2002: 53) suggests, when women's bodies are treated as a marketable resource and when the female body is viewed as capital, this is based on a male-centered logic.

The consuming body: female purchasing power

Anderson (2005) elaborates on the economic power of drug-using women when she focuses on the power of women drug users as consumers and their ability to raise finances for the purchase of goods and services which helps stimulate both the illegal and legal economies. She cites three income sources, sex-work, social transfer payments and secondary labour market employment, and contends that the capability of consuming is fundamental to personal existence and the growth of capitalist economies. Rather than look specifically at the abovementioned income sources, I want to look more generally at drug-using women as consumers of goods and services for drug use and, as Anderson (2005) contends, powerful economic actors. The realm of consumer culture in contemporary society is a site for the reproduction of social inequalities and reinforcement of normativity. (See the following chapter for a discussion on drug use and consumption.) Furthermore, consumer culture actively creates a particular kind of self which is orientated towards self-indulgence rather than self-denial and which regards the self as being of prime importance (Howson, 2004: 93–4). The consumption of drugs shares common ground and flourishes within an addictive society. While drug use may be viewed as 'criminal consumption', designated as deviant and mainly serving male interests or, as discussed earlier in Chapter 2, male, street cultural capital (Collison, 1996), the consuming body of the female drug user is able to gain competence, control and power (Murphy and Arroyo, quoted in Anderson, 2005). This is particularly true if they are able to maximize their street utility (Bretteville-Jensen, 1999: 380) and determine their optimal consumption level.

While this consuming female body is both a construction and a resource, this body is built up by various burdensome social and moral discourses, although leakages from daily domination are possible, if women are able to offer resistance in the midst of social vulnerability. For example, women and minorities are constituted politically in part by virtue of the social vulnerability of their bodies – as a site of desire and physical vulnerability, and of a publicity at once assertive and exposed (Butler, 2004: 20). Here social vulnerability can be translated into cultural adages that say: 'Drug use is anathema to women's bodies as carers and reproducers' or 'Women who consume drugs fail in their social responsibility to be the guardians of morals'. These are usual refrains emerging from these social and moral discourses.

Although female users may control economic resources, they are able to embody a productive resistance, reminding us that they are not automatons of social and institutional forces (Baker, 2000). This resistance is simultaneous with a type of performative agency that can be shared by other abject bodies in a drug-consuming space. This agency exists regardless of the fact that some women may be ill-equipped to handle the violence that is necessary to maintain security and control (Fagan, 1994) in these settings. Through the power of the biomedical discourse, drug use is not indicative of a body consuming health (Ettorre and Miles, 2001). Furthermore, for all women consuming health is a social imperative (Doyal, 2002). Nevertheless these resourceful, consuming bodies create opportunities for embodying themselves as an asset, strong and coping. While the moral outrage levelled against women drug users is one more deployment in the stigmatization of women's drug-using bodies, this can also be an occasion for these female bodies to privilege their monstrous bodies and performativities of disgust. Here the consuming body of the female drug user creates space for an imaginative form of femininity: at least her consumption provides a certain amount of power, albeit this power is defined by the extent to which it supports male structures.

The female labouring body: women subsidizing men's use

Related to the above consuming body is the female labouring body. In discussing sources of women's economic power, Anderson (2005) notes that subsidizing male drug users, their consumption of drugs, sustenance needs, and lifestyles is a core activity for women drug users. Anderson (2005: 385) says that few studies have addressed the vulnerable position of the male addict and the empowered position of the female sex worker and/or drug user in providing for him. Instead, previous work has constructed this as another form of women's powerlessness and exploitation – for example, men force women into sex work to financially support their habits.

In this context, given that the female body has no stable history, the valuation put on this body has been constant only in so far as it has been consistently less than the value given to the male body (Shildrick, 1997: 22). This is especially true in the drugs field where women's needs are reconstructed as risks and viewed as undeserving of the status 'victim' or even 'citizen' (Malloch, 2004). The implication is that in order to see clearly the value or resource of gendered bodies – especially drug-using, female labouring bodies – we must look at these bodies in relation. Thus when women financially support men's drug-using activities, their bodies become 'relational resources' regardless of whether their relationships are marked by risky behaviours (for example, unsafe sex, drug use, injecting, victimization, violence, betrayal, exploitation, and so on).

Both female and male users engage in risk relationships and love and intimacy may play a large part in managing these embodied relationships. In order for women to be successful as labouring relational bodies, they need to appreciate the forms of difficult embodiments and complex, gendered rules of engagement in their intimate liaisons and social identities. For example, let's look at drug using, female sex workers. These women are confronted with not only the risks associated with work relationships but also changing drug fashions (that is, from crack cocaine, to powder cocaine, to ecstasy, and so on) (Green, Day and Ward, 2000). These women need to be aware of the risks and benefits associated with these changing drug fashions and the variety of ways different drugs feature in worker, client, manager and dealer relationships in the 'sex industry'. While some drug-using women may thrive economically in this environment, others may become increasingly desperate and find their marketability and bargaining power so reduced that they accept a fraction of the money they once received for their services (Willies and Rushforth, 2003). Anna Green, Sophie Day and Helen Ward (2000) found it was difficult for female sex workers to separate professional, work-related from recreational drug use. They experienced their bodies as 'occupational resources', shaped by different relationships between 'working' and 'private' partners, similar to other women who relied on their bodies to produce income (Evans et al., 2002). Here, drugs and risky sex cut across both the public and the private boundaries of work and leisure. As labouring bodies supporting partners, female users of all ages, sexual orientations, classes and ethnicities find that these bodies turn out to be relational investments – useful physical capital or resources (Bordo, 1993a) similar to other non-drug-using women.

The female body 'in commerce': dealing drugs

While drug-dealing activities may be the most coveted jobs in the illicit drug economy, the number of women involved in drug selling, their location in the pecking order and whether or not they are gaining ground in relation to men remain burning issues (Anderson, 2005) in the drugs field. In this context, the gendered drug-using bodies that we come into contact with and conceptualize are at all times seen to be mediated by constructs, associations and images of a cultural nature. For instance, biology is important in so far as it is contextualized by culture. The body itself is contextualized by difference – race, gender, ethnicity, sexual orientation and class.

When women drug users become engaged in dealing drugs, their bodies are inscribed by culture in the commercial world through the business of doing drugs. Barbara Denton and Pat O'Malley (1999) describe how the illicit drug market is fragmentary and competitive, lending itself to small business entrepreneurs. They contend that this small business structure may make it more practicable for women to succeed in this illicit economy and, furthermore, that the lack of a clear authority structure and the capacity to absorb new dealers provides fewer barriers for women dealers to overcome. This research is instructive in that we learn how those in women dealer's family networks become a stable and reliable operational base for women to be successful as drug entrepreneurs and financially resourceful. These female bodies embrace drug dealing while resisting full-blown embodiment in the circle of kith and kin. Their deviant embodiment evidences a movement or type of fluidity between disciplined, fiscally focused bodies and apparently undisciplined bodies shaped by families, properties and patriarchal interests. But as Fiona Hutton (2005: 547) points out, patriarchal interests operate in the world of drug dealing and women dealers cannot be seen as operating independently of hegemonic masculinity and its relationship with subcultural capital.

In this area, the embodiment discourse can show that it makes a difference whose drug dealing bodies we are talking about. In the past, the standard core of the body in commerce, whether drug using or not, was usually a White, male, middle-class body, passing as the norm for all. This discourse on the body and drugs should expose the fact that gender, race and ethnicity, as well as class, make a difference. More importantly, it establishes the fact that there are differential accounts of female and male agency, and that female embodiment in the form of drug dealing is incorporated easily in the disciplinary machinery of the illicit drug economy, particularly when this embodied activity is supported by intimacy, trust and primary relationships (Denton and O Malley, 1999) – all resources that have been culturally feminized.

Whether or not drug dealing is a corporeal style, the dealing female body gives us insights into how restrictive masculinist assumptions about the character of the procedures and skills involved in drug dealing can be overturned. Nevertheless we must be cautious in assuming that women have greater participation than ever before in the drug distribution business, as noted above. Lisa Maher and David Dixon (1999) show that women are often recruited into drug sales because the police are less likely to search them. However, once police are on to this scheme women are not as likely to be recruited to sell drugs (Friedman and Alicia, 2001). Here the gaze of the law (Moran, 2001) enacted by the corporality of policing in the drugs world is organized around masculinist assumptions about which bodies should deal drugs. But when female bodies are recruited into this activity and become bona fide dealers, there is a chance that their defiance of traditional expectations may remain invisible, while at the same time their legitimacy as dealers becomes somewhat tenuous, if not denied.

Whether or not dealing drugs is an empowering embodied experience (Friedman and Alicia, 2001) for these women, involvement in this core activity will inevitably have corporeal consequences for significant others around them. For example, this is demonstrated when Marilyn, a forty-year-old dealer interviewed by Friedman and Alicia (2001: 135) says:

> There was this thing with the Filas [expensive name-brand shoes]. I explained to them [her children] either Mom uses, deals drugs and you have Filas or I don't use, I'm in treatment and you have Payless shoes. I told them you have a choice . . .
> use, don't use
> deal, treatment
> Filas, Payless
> . . . They chose the Payless shoes. They wanted me around.

Perhaps Marilyn's reflections point to a communicative body (Frank, 1995) which we discussed in a previous context (see Chapter 2). Although Arthur Frank (1995: 150) uses this notion in the context of ill or wounded bodies, we can envisage female drug-using bodies in this way – as communicative bodies – that is, bodies needing empathy and a relationship/s in which one understands oneself as requiring listening from another. Marilyn, the dealer mentioned above, gets empathy from her children. The discourse of care is placed within the language of survival as her caring is rendered both instrumental and contingent (Frank, 1995: 150).

A critique of 'core activities' theorizing

Although Anderson's (2005) ideas on core activities are novel, they can be criticized from a feminist point of view and I will offer four criticisms. First, two core activities hint at a consensus view of women's roles. Secondly, a basic assumption of Anderson's work is that skills acquired in the illegal drug culture can be transferred automatically to conventional society. Thirdly, she does not question women's access to power as through relations. Lastly, the notion of women's abject status is not problematized. Let us look at each of these criticisms in turn. My main aim in offering these criticisms is to demonstrate that a feminist embodiment perspective can be seen as a necessary corrective to what Anderson offers.

First, in my interpretation of Anderson's (2005) core activities, I see that two activities – women's control of the household and women's consuming or using their purchasing power – hint at normative processes which are required of most, if not all women. Indeed, these processes are the effect of regulatory practices that seek to render the female bodies who engage in these processes as performing heteronormative activities, viewed as 'standard' for all women. Of course, subsidizing men's drug use and using purchasing power for drug consumption are not perceived as 'normal' activities for women. But supporting men in this way may be taken for granted as it is 'in conventional society' when women perform similar 'supporting' activities in their relationships with their male partners. Thus implicit in these activities is a legitimating and legitimation process, a rubber stamping of the need for women to support men. Simply, this view reflects a type of safety-valve theory in the drugs field in which women's emotional and physical care-giving is viewed not only as securing psychological benefits for individual men but also as shoring up the patriarchal system as a whole (see Bartky, 1990, pp. 105–7 for a full discussion of this 'safety-valve theory'). Nevertheless, this is not meant to deny the fact that women drug users can be active and independent participants in the drugs world, with diverse lifestyles and experiences (Morgan and Joe, 1996).

Secondly, Anderson implies that the transferable skills gained by their participation in these core activities are important for women if and when they re-enter conventional society. Yes, it is important for women drug users to be able to convert their 'deviant' drug-using lifestyles to more conventional ones and to reassign their responsibility, management of risk and strength to conventional actions. A more apt question would be, 'Do these types of activities establish a legitimate basis for making citizenship claims?' We must ensure that the notion of core activities makes room for a level of resistance, incoherence and instability in finding female empowerment through alternative activities such as pleasure-seeking, self-determination in promoting harm reduction and self-governance. While Anderson argues that this transition is needed in articulating a link between mainstream and deviant contexts, women are not on a level playing field vis-à-vis men. It is their skills, not men's which need to be seen as transferable. Furthermore the domestic sites of women's work remain outside and are subservient to what Smith (1990: 17–18) calls the governing conceptual mode of our society, in which men, not women dominate.

Thirdly, Anderson (2005: 374) is very keen to move away from what she calls a 'pathology narrative' and emphasizes the variety of ways women users acquire 'money capital', becoming powerful economic actors. She does not interrogate why in her schema women's access to power is usually, if not mainly relational (to heterosexual, if not always White men) and certainly not structural. Whatever way one looks at her women, they are not only second class but are empowered by being second class. Most importantly, in my view this demonstrates that she does not question the actual lived reality of many women. For example, it is important to recognize how female bodies are being pressed into the service of men and money capital generally and in the illicit drug economy, specifically. However, these explanations based on work, localization and marked bodies need to make room for conceptions of fragmented gendered embodied subjects in homes, workplaces, drugs markets and public arenas which are constantly being coded and dispersed in infinite ways with grave consequences for women (see Haraway, 1991: 163). Simply, we need to ensure that our theorizing allows for a level of visible opposition and anti-oppressive approaches which are necessary for women's survival.

Lastly, the notion of women's abject status is not problematized. Simply, women in Anderson's view who engage in these core activities are theorized in term of local investment, as well as strategic defence strategies. There is little if any awareness of how these female bodies themselves have become abject, monstrous objects to be disassembled and reassembled and coded into diseased objects of knowledge and sites of intervention (see Urla and Terry, 1995). By focusing on gender, Anderson perpetuates the opposition of male and female which is inherently heterosexist and does not allow for other sexualities to emerge (Brook, 1999: 5). Furthermore, related to this lack is the obscuring of how both sexualized and racialized bodies become sites of intervention in the drug-using world.

The above demonstrates clearly that there are problems, conflicts and difficulties in defining women's relationship to drug use as a feminist issue. Offering new feminist embodiment approaches is important because it pushes the boundaries of our theory-making at a time when we need other raced, classed and gendered bodies to be included in our theory making.

Embodiment, women and drugs

While the construction of 'the body' is an effect of endless circulation of power and knowledge, the female drug-using body, as we now sense, provides the focus for regulatory techniques practised on an individual, perceived as a shameful, unfeminine and irresponsible female – a monstrous, abject body. As we have seen, a major premise supporting women drug users' engagement in core activities is that the female body is normalized as life-giver and reproducer. It is almost as if this valorisation is taken as a biological given.

Today we recognize the importance of women's core activities in shaping women's experience in the illegal drug economy. But we must also envisage woman's drug use as a type of female embodiment constructed and disciplined in relationship to others and her reproductive body (Campbell, 1999). Within the context of medical science, the symbol of the age of biopower is the reproductive body, the body of a woman capable of and/or in fact producing babies under the benevolent guise of medicine. As I noted in Chapter 2, biopower is all about the power of normativity over the living organism.

In this sense, modernity's marking of female bodies as reproductive has been a crucial way in which biopower produces and normalizes female bodies to serve prevailing gender relations of dominance and subordination, and significantly this happens in the drugs field through the sorts of assumptions we make about women's involvement in core activities, as well as reproduction (the latter issue will be discussed further in Chapter 6). Women's bodies have been inscribed by reproduction and the discourse of reproduction has been shaped by women's bodies. Female bodies have been set up alongside nature and irrationality, while male bodies have been the stronghold of reason.

With the rise of Cartesian dualism, there has been a denigration of bodies generally with a masculinist assault on nature and all things feminine – thus the notion of monstrous bodies emerges as representing women, a fact which, as we have seen, is missing from the abovementioned 'core activities' theorizing. As women's bodies, both non-drug-using and drug-using, are pressed into the service of reproduction, their social agency becomes created, defined and valued by how well they reproduce. And of course, as we already know for drug users, reproduction is a problematic issue (Murphy and Rosenbaum, 1999).

As we develop our feminist embodiment approaches to women and drugs, we should recall that the distinctiveness of being a female drug-using body is neither stable nor secure. The female drug-using body is constituted fragilely over time, instituted in various public and private spaces and established with others through stylized, repetitive performances of 'deviant' social acts and 'core activities'. While the notion of drug using may be applied to women drug users as a mark of cultural difference this is not a full picture. We need to understand and include in our analyses how female embodiment shapes the opportunities for successful social, cultural and financial engagement in domestic, consuming, labouring and dealing spaces. The message here is that in envisaging women drug users' attempts at stability in the physical and temporal spaces constructed around and through their bodies, we acknowledge the precariousness of the act of taking drugs itself. Alongside this acknowledgment is an awareness of women drug users who may continually resist embodied attributes, gendered identities and oppressive roles, targeting them as more domesticated, deviant, more reproductive and less fiscally able than men.

In contemporary sociology, the body, as a central element in the construction of the social, has become the template upon which cultural identities are fashioned and through which emotions are played out. In the context of the gendering and problematic nature of drug use, the task of the feminist sociologist is to bear witness to this form of embodied oppression through a gendered lens. This body should be placed at the core of our political struggles and theoretical work. When will we develop a morality of the female drug-using body that is attentive to diversity, discontent, disgust, deviance and conflict?

Given that the biomedical and legal discourses on the body have become embedded in contemporary cultures, we should position bodies centrally in the sociology of drug use. Yet those working in the field of biomedicine, criminal justice and law continue to devise ways of transforming the boundaries of drug-using bodies. Indeed, there is a powerful desire to classify forms of deviance, locate them in biology and patrol them in wider social spaces. Since the nineteenth century (Urla and Terry, 1995), bodies have become marked and social relations organized in terms of deviant and conforming bodies. Through an awareness of the complexities of the workings of gender, embodiment and power we are able to contextualize and understand the conditions and experiences of living, drug-using communities of gendered, embodied subjects. (See also the discussion in Chapter 6 on the 'somatic territorializing of deviance'.)

Specifically, when we look at the social and cultural processes marking the boundaries between drug-using and non-drug-using bodies we see the normative discourses which shape abnormal or deviant bodies as distinct from normal ones. In this chapter I have also demonstrated how Anderson's (2005) core activities can be applied to a feminist embodiment perspective, notwithstanding the limitations in this type of 'core activities' theorizing. By making women's bodies central in the discourse about core activities, acknowledging discourses which target them and allowing space for the emergence of a communicative body, I have hopefully exposed the female body as a subject to and of truths about drugs. With this in mind, I focus in the next three chapters specifically on different types of embodiment for female drug users.

5
Drug-Consuming Bodies

> They are all in trouble today, the mass-circulation magazines,
> vying fiercely with each other and television to deliver more
> and more millions of women who will buy the things their
> advertisers sell. Does this frantic race force the men who
> make the images to see women only as thing-buyers? Does it
> force them to compete finally in emptying women's minds
> of human thought? . . .
>
> Betty Friedan (1963: 58)

The sociological field of consumption

As noted in Chapter 1, I ask in this and the following two
chapters the question, 'How can we develop a feminist embodiment approach to drug use?' and look at some of the different types
of embodiments that are on offer to drug-using women. Already
in the previous chapter I used the notion of the consuming body
to demonstrate women drug users' bodies as being the embodiment of female purchasing power in the world of illegal drug use
via Tammy Anderson's (2005) 'core activities' theorizing. In that
context I looked at drug-using women as consumers of goods and
services and strong economic actors and, mostly, at their bodies as
resources. I want in this chapter to embed the notion of consuming
bodies in the contemporary material culture of illegal drugs. In
consumer society, all of us, whether drug using or not, find ourselves
constantly constituted in face to face interactions. This is mainly
because consumerism and the mass market have blurred the exterior

marks of social and personal difference: our lives have become stylized while our bodies have been commodified (Turner, 1996: 122–4).

In looking in this chapter at what I call the sociological field of consumption, I want to review features of modern consumer culture with regard to drug-consuming bodies. When looking at this sociological field of consumption I draw upon the work of British sociologists Celia Lury and Mike Featherstone who have written extensively on consumption. On the one hand, Celia Lury (1996) provides a clear outline of the distinctive characteristics of contemporary consumer culture, while on the other hand, Mike Featherstone (1982, 1991) focuses on consumption vis-à-vis urbanization and the body in consumer culture. I also draw upon the work of sociologist Hugh MacKay (1997: 10) whose approach (and that of his colleagues) is somewhere between the liberated, pleasurable consumer and the critique of mass culture approach to consumption.

The chapter is divided into three interrelated discussions. First, I will look at sociological work (Lury, 1996) which outlines distinctive characteristics of contemporary consumer culture related to the availability of consumer goods; sites for purchase and consumption; political organization of consumers and consumer illnesses. I offer a discussion of these factors with special reference to drug consumption. Secondly, I discuss urbanization and consumption (Featherstone, 1991) and the body in consumer culture (Featherstone, 1982). Here I attempt to link these conceptualizations to gender and drug use. Thirdly, I attempt to extend the notion of consuming body to 'consumption themes' (MacKay, 1997) involving the balance between creativity and restraint; the interrelationship between consumption and production; the situated character of everyday practices; the broad range of consumption practices and the spatial dimension of consumption. All themes, as we shall see, have relevance for gendered drug-consuming bodies. My assumption, which underpins all the discussions in this chapter, is that revisioning women and drugs through the lens of consumption will not only help to challenge obsolete ways of thinking about female drug use but also push our minds to consider the ordinariness of drug consumption for some, if not most users.

Drug-consuming bodies to drug-communicative bodies?

In her book *Consumer Culture*, Celia Lury (1996: 4) attempts to classify what is distinctive about consumer culture as a specific form of material culture in Euro-American societies. She puts forward the thesis that consumer culture is best defined as a process of stylization. Furthermore, Lury (1996: 29–36) endeavours to consider the special characteristics of contemporary material culture and, in doing so, she outlines what she refers to as the 15 distinctive features which characterize modern consumption. While she sees these features as diverse and not all equally important features of modern life, she asserts that all features are related to the rapid increase in consumer demand associated with modern industrial societies. While there is no space in this chapter to look in detail at each of the 15 features she discusses, I want to focus on four features which can be linked specifically to contemporary drug consumption. These include: (i) availability of a large (and constantly increasing) number and range of consumer goods; (ii) an increase in sites for purchase and consumption; (iii) political organization by and of consumers; and (iv) the increasing visibility of so-called consumer illnesses linked to pathologies or maladies of the will. Overall this discussion demonstrates how the realm of consumer culture in contemporary society with special reference to drug consumption provides not only sites for the reproduction of social inequalities but also for reinforcements of normativity and distinct moral values related to drug-consumption practices. Let us look briefly at each feature in turn and make links with the drugs field and gender, respectively.

Availability of a large (and constantly increasing) number and range of drugs to be consumed

Regarding this first feature of consumer culture with special reference to drug consumption, we look specifically at the availability and array of drugs. We know that an increasing range of different types of drugs is consumed in contemporary societies (Barton, 2003). Globally, drugs have different social meanings in various cultures (Knipe, 1995) and from a cross-cultural perspective, public opinions and societal attitudes towards the same drugs or addictive substances with similar properties can vary significantly. Simply, not all drug use is stigmatized consistently across cultures (Coomber and South, 2004a).

Each year new drugs hit the illegal (Ramsay and Partridge, 1999) and legal drugs (Wren, 2005) markets, fuelling different types of drug careers and lifestyles and, as we saw earlier, when women become involved in drug markets they may triumph as dealers (Denton and O'Malley, 1999). As prominence of any particular drug may shift in urban street markets, for example from heroin to cocaine, this sequence of events rules the relations between the gendered, racialized body and the market experience.

Shifts in drug prominence may enable further market movements with the result that Black and ethnic minority women are able to embody successful drug-selling careers (Fagan, 1994; 1995). Furthermore, involvement in the illicit drug market may be experienced by some women as a form of positive embodiment, bringing economic independence, self-esteem, professional pride and a sense of ethics (Morgan and Joe, 1996) to their deviant lives. Here shifts in the availability and array of drugs may allow women or indeed men to embody roles of drug intermediaries. But one's economic status will consistently set limits on any drug user's participation in drug consumption or their practical freedom to exercise choice concerning what drug to consume (see Lury, 1996: 6).

An increase in sites for purchase and consumption of drugs

An obvious link with the increasing availability and array of drugs is an increase in sites for drug purchase and drug consumption, the second feature of consumption I will discuss in this context. In the illicit drugs culture there have traditionally been public and private spaces – shooting galleries, rooms, homes, cinemas, prisons, public toilets, abandoned cars, streets and street corners, clinics for drug users, pharmacies, and so on – where people can purchase and consume their drugs. In terms of this spatial dimension of drug consumption, less usual spaces, such as phone boxes (see 'Council to dig up phone boxes – the new crack houses', *Druglink*, 2004, 19, 5: 2) and legally sanctioned environments such as drug consumption rooms (Roberts, Klein and Trace, 2004) have become of late visible sites for drug consumption. In recent years, cyberspace or the Internet provides a ripe area for accessing or developing knowledge of sources for supplying drugs, as well as learning about the range and diversity of drugs and their effects (Dearling, 1999: 136).

Of course, the workings of gender in this mix are often obscured given that the sorts of resource acquisition strategies that some drug-using women employ to obtain and consume their drugs tend to be shaped by economies of high risk (Miller and Neagius, 2002). Very often for some of these women economic deprivation inter-acts with their risky consumption and coalesces with their chosen consumption sites, their HIV status and other perceived risks, such as incarceration, homelessness, loss of children.

Over the years, there has been expanded participation in informal drug economies or democratization in the social and economic contexts where drugs are bought and sold. However, these sorts of democratized opportunities have not extended to women (Jacobs and Miller, 1998). In effect, while drug-using women may be actively aware of sites for drug purchase and drug consumption, unlike men, these women may not have full access to these contexts. Thus, regu-lation and control of one's own drug consumption may represent for some women the only immediate area within which a female drug-consuming body is able to express governance and authority. Also, even if a woman is a dealer and perhaps more aware than other women users of sites for purchase and consumption, her governance and authority will be limited as she needs to battle to secure her consumer product at a reasonable price in the hegemonic mascu-line, consumer culture in which she operates in her business dealings (Hutton, 2005).

Political organization by and of drug consumers

With regard to the political organizing of drug users, we know that national drug users' networks exist in countries such as Canada, the Netherlands, Russia, Thailand, Australia and Denmark. These drug users' networks exist to protect the interests of drug users, mainly in their consumption of treatment services as well as, in some instances, the provision of drugs (see Derks, Hoekstra and Kaplan, 1996). Perhaps the best known drug users' advocacy group is Amsterdam's Junkiebond in the Netherlands. This group's members have been concerned with protecting the human rights of users and identifying the risks that injection drug users pose to themselves and others (Van Ameijden, 1992; Buning et al., 1986). There have also been moves afoot in the UK to build up service user groups (Chequer, 2006; Brain, 2006) as distinct consumers, demanding services which value dignity and self-respect for every customer who comes through the door for help (Shapiro, 2005).

While the political organization of drug consumers, whether as users or consumers of services, is important, we need to ask a series of questions. Who benefits from these political actions? Are drug users really able to create their own political interests? How will we account for the fact that consumption patterns of drug users vary by gender (Bretteville-Jensen, 1999)? What about women consumers, given that gender differences in drug users' take up of treatment services exist with more women than men at a distinct disadvantage (Callaghan and Cunningham, 2002; Green et al., 2002; Arfken et al., 2002)? What are we able to say about the needs of Black and ethnic minority women who as drug consumers can be excluded from both the legal and illegal economic systems (Cross et al., 2001)? These questions help to sharpen our focus and remind us that gender, race and ethnicity need to be considered as important components of the culture of drug consumption, as well as drug consumer politics.

Here, while an anti-foundationalist or non-essentialist view of the body emphasizes the changeable, malleable and contingent characteristic of embodiment in consumer societies (Turner, 1996: 5), racialized, gendered and classed drug-consuming bodies may be limited in their engagement with drug-consumer politics, if not excluded very often from these politics altogether.

The increasing visibility of drug use as a consumer illness linked to maladies of the will

With regard to our fourth feature of drug consumption, Celia Lury (1996: 36) mentions specifically the increasing visibility of so-called consumer illnesses linked to pathologies or maladies of the will. In that context she mentions Eva Sedgwick's (1994) work *Tendencies*. Out of all of the features of consumer culture Lury mentions, this one has perhaps the most relevance for looking at drug use and embodied drug consumption. This is because this feature directs our attention immediately to drug-consuming bodies and the moral effects of this type of consumption on contemporary society.

For example, as a result of the cultural shaping of 'new' categories of addiction, such as drug addict, food addict, exercise addict

(Terry, Szabo and Griffiths, 2004), shopaholic, sex addict, workaholic (Griffiths, 2005), internet addiction (Kaltiala-Heino, Lintonen and Rimpelä, 2004), even addiction to gasoline or petrol (à la President George Bush), and so on, we come to understand how the discourse of free will becomes embedded in contemporary consumer culture. Through an intermixing of the 'epidemic of addiction paradigm' with what Sedgwick (1994: 135) refers to as the consumer phase of international capitalism, material, fleshy bodies become sites of addiction. These sites of addiction exhibit a deficiency – of a 'healthy' free will – when consuming one's 'choice' of addiction.

In this way, epidemics of the will such as drug addiction reinforce a type of normativity. More importantly, the 'epidemic' of drug addiction which is all about the ingestion of a 'foreign' substance becomes an overarching and powerful abstraction which governs the narrative relations between the body and the addiction experience (Sedgwick, 1994: 131). Here the main point of Sedgwick's argument is that consuming bodies, whatever foreign substance or behaviour they consume, are characteristically imbued with free will. Moreover these consuming bodies are charged with ethical value, depending upon *what* they consume, *the compulsions* behind their everyday consumption and *the success* of expressing their natural needs over and above their artificial desires (for example, addictions).

For drug users, their consuming bodies are seen to embody a compulsion to consume dangerous, foreign substances. Embodied tensions are bound to emerge. For example, in the current discursive constructions of consumer capitalism, the power of drug users' free will is always already contaminated by the 'truth' of her/his compulsion, while the power attached to her/his acknowledged compulsion such as drug use is always already contaminated by the 'truth' of her/his free will (Sedgwick, 1994: 141–2). Plainly, these drug-consuming bodies cannot escape the incessant charging of bodies with the habitual and regulatory regimes of medicine, law and, more importantly, morality, as we shall see.

Within this liberal humanist discourse and through the lens of gender, class and race, this picture becomes clearer, yet more complicated. We see men and women, young and old, Black and White, advantaged and disadvantaged, and so on, as being equally entitled to become responsible moral agents. Yet the ideal construction of a responsible moral agent exercising her/his option of free will or consent is deeply problematic on a series of linked levels, material and discursive, not the least of which is sexual (Shidrick, 1997: 83) difference (and I would add, racial difference).

Here, in a society based on normative, privileged, White, male standards, women, particularly Black and ethnic minority women or indigenous women, are not considered fully rational in the first place (Shildrick, 1997: 85). Thus, in order to challenge these norms, the bodies of all drug users need to be mobilized into an ethical economy (Shidrik, 2001: 171) in which classed, gendered, racialized and aged specificities are in communion or unity with the differences between us all. Simply we collapse the category 'difference'. Thus far, this may be impossible in our consumer cultures, including those bound up with drugs.

In looking at Lury's four features vis-à-vis drug consumption, I would contend that the drug-consuming body should become visible more as a communicative body than as a chaotic body, which is the other against which the communicative body defines itself (Frank, 1995: 104). This means that rather than becoming victims to dominating bodies which make them the object of their force (Frank, 1995: 104, 154), drug-consuming bodies as communicative bodies become open to communion with others and learn from their own and other's suffering, as well as successes. In effect, drug-consuming bodies are able to offer themselves up to public consumption and allow themselves to be assessed on the adequacy of their performance of selves in a drug-consuming as well as drug-moralizing society. This type of cultural 'offering up' implies a distinct questioning of the boundary between public and private. It implies a questioning of the boundaries between staged performances (that is, public consumption of drugs) as a separate sphere and the everyday enactment or performance of self (that is, self-governance of one's body as a drug consumer) (Brook, 1999: 113). In this context, the notion of performance questions the authenticity of what is being offered up, as well as the 'true' identity of the 'performer' in consumer culture. Simply, the idea of performance implies an ethical gap between what we see (that is, drug-consuming bodies) and what we think might be their invisible origin (that is, an unhealthy free will) (see Brook, 1999: 113).

Translating the above sorts of ideas to the drug-consuming body means that we are able to envisage drug-consuming activities as integrated with other social and cultural activities. Also, these ideas emphasize that while drug consumption may involve an exchange of benefits between people, this type of cultural consumption does not necessarily exhibit the sort of physical control commensurate with the display of a hyper-efficient performing self in consumer cultures (Shilling, 2005: 2).

However, female drug-consuming bodies face unique circumstances that are indisputably gendered regardless of whether or not they may create staged performances to camouflage drug sales and consumption (Jacobs and Miller, 1998). Again, we are faced here with the incessant structural reality that racialized, gendered and classed bodies are often limited in their engagement with the consumer culture of illegal drugs as a specific form of material culture in contemporary social life.

Drug consumption vis-à-vis urbanization

In the chapter 'City cultures and postmodern lifestyles' in his book *Consumer culture and postmodernism*, Mike Featherstone (1991: 96) focuses on transformations in lifestyles and city cultures, cultural specialists, such as interpreters, carriers and promoters of a range of cultural goods and experiences, and the perceptions of those goods and experiences as significant, meaningful and worthy of consumption. In that context Featherstone (1991: 96) examines three factors which point to the ways in which the cultures of cities and urban lifestyles have become what he calls, 'thematized': (i) the notion of cultural centres; (ii) how consumption is mediated by diverse cultural images; and (iii) the pursuit of lifestyle and stylization of life. Similar to the above discussion on Lury's ideas, I intend in the following to translate some of these ideas into the drugs field with special reference to gendered embodiment.

In his work Featherstone (1991: 99–100) contends that there is an assumption that particular cities are cultural centres which exude cultural capital and are the centres of cultural consumption as well as general consumption. Within this framework, our postmodern cities appear as urban spaces in which people who move through these spaces are able to celebrate the fact that the urban iconography of clothes, bodies, faces, and so on, are artificial, opaque and depthless. This is in the sense that this urban iconography cannot be decoded in order to offer access to some fundamental sense of truth.

Significantly, urban consumers revel in this experience. Although Featherstone focuses specifically on cities that represent centres of cultural reproduction, as well as house mass culture industries such as fashion, popular music, tourism, leisure, and so on, his key notions can be converted to a deeper understanding of how drug-consuming bodies occupy urban spaces.

Here we see that with regard to drug consumption there are assumptions surrounding specific cities or metropolises, such as Liverpool, Glasgow, Barcelona, Moscow, Warsaw, New Haven and Rome. These urban centres are where, on the one hand, the illegal economy of drug production and consumption is able to flourish and, on the other hand, where many drug-related deaths are recorded (Davoli, 1997). Nevertheless it is within these drug conurbations that drug users as supposedly de-centred subjects are provided with amorphous and diffuse drug experiences, if not gratification from drugs.

While the urban club culture in 1990s Britain epitomized this sort of subjectivity, the significance of clubs was the direct personal experience of the power and potential of collective mobilization, of being part of a community, regardless of its form and direction (Measham, Aldridge and Parker, 2001: 30). It was and is in these and other drug-consuming contexts that de-centred subjects have a greater capacity to engage in a 'controlled de-control' of the emotions and explore immediate sensations and affective experiences formerly regarded as threatening or needing to be kept at bay (Featherstone, 1991: 101). In postmodern cities, all sorts of drugs can become an object of the drug consumer's gaze. As a result, different 'drug tribes' are able to emerge. I liken these drug tribes to Featherstone's (1991:101) postmodern tribes, the temporary emotional communities in which intense moments of ecstasy, empathy and affectual immediacy are experienced and where masses of people come together.

In this context, Henderson's (1999: 43) female drug tribe can be seen as the temporary emotional community in which drugs were one of a wide range of illicit cultural products. It was the space where female drug users composed a lifestyle and through which they made sense of themselves within the broader context of the gendered social world. Here, the pursuit of a drug-stylized lifestyle can be seen to represent a gendered presentation of self linked with the aestheticization of everyday life (Featherstone, 1991). Simply, through the performance of the self, one's life can be shaped aesthetically.

For drug users, this type of consumer stylization becomes embedded in practices of drug consumption that go beyond an instrumental, rational calculus to an emotional experience and affective investment in a drug-using lifestyle. While the idea of a female drug tribe may, at first glance, be seen to have a distinct British flavour, female drug tribes exist in, for example, Europe, Canada and the United States. However, in the consumption cultures of drug use in these countries, it appears that it is easier for researchers (see Campbell, 1999; Boyd and Faith, 1999; Stocco et al., 2000; Hedrich, 2000) to emphasize a criminal-justice and/or treatment perspective rather than a cultural, consumption one.

The picture of postmodern consumption that Featherstone paints is one honed by images of contemporary popular culture in fashion, the Internet, music, CDs, videos, drugging, dancing, clubbing, stylizations of urban consumption and imageries of fun, chaos and celebration. But social exclusion is a fundamental part of general consumption and the specific drug-consumption landscape.

Here, in an attempt to resolve the tension between being de-centred subjects and experiencing structural exclusion, drug users may participate in a variety of street crimes – but not all drug users (Allen, 2006). Particularly, male drug users may take refuge in an urban drug economy and celebrate a misogynist predatory street culture that normalizes gang rape, sexual conquest and paternal abandonment (Bourgois, 1996). On the other hand, women's consumption in these contexts is often shaped by violence (Erickson et al., 2000; Martin and Bryant, 2001), partner abuse (Wilson Cohn, Strauss and Falkin, 2002), sexually transmitted diseases (Latka et al., 2001), poverty (Vaarwerk and Gaal) and homelessness (Belcher et al., 2001), other, less aesthetic sides of the celebratory urban culture of drug consumption. Furthermore, regardless of the ethnic composition of the above metropolises where drug consumption takes place, the development of these cities rests on a hierarchal system of dualisms between White, privileged male and coloured, classed, female, in which the former bodies are privileged over the latter.

Unfortunately, this hierarchal sense of dualisms is not only missing from Featherstone's analysis of postmodern cities but also the majority of drug research work. As a result, we are left with little, if any idea of gender or race embodiments vis-à-vis general consumption and, in turn, drug consumption in major drug conurbations.

This is with the exception of the perceived wisdom in the field that the governing discourse on drug consumption reflects gender, race and economic biases and, at times, structural inequalities.

The drug-using body in consumer culture

Staying with Mike Featherstone's (1982) work and his interest in consumer culture, I turn now to his classic article 'The body in consumer culture' and continue to make links with the drug field. In Featherstone's (1982: 170) view, within contemporary culture all sorts of cultural products presented in advertisements, television, cinema, bill boards, and so on, provide a proliferation of stylized images of the body.

Aggressively, consumer culture generates a distinct kind of self which is orientated towards pleasure, hedonism and self-indulgence rather than self-effacement and denial. Consumer culture latches on to the prevailing self-preservationist body conceptions encouraging individuals to adopt instrumental strategies to combat bodily decline and decay. Furthermore, consumer culture unites all of these conceptions with the idea of the body as a vehicle of self-expression and pleasure. For Featherstone (1982: 186) the body in consumer culture has become secularized and self-preservation of this self-same body depends upon the preservation of the body within a culture in which the body is the passport to all that is good in life.

Within consumer culture, a performing self emerges which places greater emphasis upon appearance, display and management of impressions (Featherstone, 1982: 187). Yet consumer culture is not merely about bodily performance, entertainment or display. Consumer culture operates on two broad levels – it provides a wealth of images designed to incite needs and desires and it is based on and helps to change the material arrangements of social space and, consequently, the whole field of social interactions (Featherstone, 1982: 192).

Looking at these ideas through the lens of drug use, we see that illegal drugs are cultural products which do not exemplify good or moral embodiment and consumption. Furthermore, drug consumption may be seen as helping deterioration and decay of the body which suggests that, for the drug consumer, bodily and behavioural change through rehabilitation is perceived by the experts as always a necessary experience prior to reengagement with consumer society (Chacksfield, 2002). On the other hand, drug consumption does not fit easily into the self-expression and pleasure nexus. The notion of the drug-using body as a vehicle of self-expression and pleasure is often hidden, if not denied. Indeed, the governing mentalities surrounding drug policy envisage drug users as non-productive and undeserving citizens. In particular, women drug users are seen to lack self-governance (Campbell, 1999: 917).

If drug consumption can be seen as part of an oppositional cultural response to mainstream culture (Koester, Anderson and Hoffer, 1999: 2148), this response needs to be seen as an embodied response – an integral part of an individual's corporeal identity. Nevertheless the drug-consuming body is the secularized body *in extremis*. Ironically, the very fact that this drug-consuming body is deeply profane separates it from other 'secularized' consuming bodies. Here we see that the embodied action of consuming an illegal drug is viewed as the self-harming rather than self-preserving of one's body. In this way, a drug-consuming body is seen to reject a culture in which the body is the means to all that is decent and moral in life. As far as the performing self is concerned, the ritual performance of taking illegal drugs is located in a domain of deviant indulgence seen as deserving moral derision and social scorn. This is over and above the fact that illusions of hedonism are generated within consumer society (Featherstone, 1982: 186) and good forms of calculating hedonism and cultural indulgence can replace asceticism for any disciplined body.

In this context, Langman (2003: 224) contends that there are episodic expressions, anti-structures or liminal sites of resistance, inversion and repudiation where social norms can be flaunted and where submerged identities and tabooed desires are expressed. These episodic expressions, such as carnivals in Rio, American football games and extreme body modifications, such as body piercing and tattooing, serve to maintain social stability through controlled violations of the cultural order.

Interestingly enough, the ritual performance of consuming a cultural product such as an illegal drug may be a form of resistance but within the governing discourse on drugs this action is not seen as maintaining social stability or given the status of a controlled infringement or sanctioned deviance. Drug use is plainly and simply deviant, wrong or off beam under Western culture's moral searchlight. Drug consumption becomes a personal and public disease. It is the paradigmatic social malady which not only conveys the infiltration of one's body with dangerous foreign substances but also evidences the breakdown of self-control and discipline as well as the embodiment of immorality and appalling health.

On the one hand, consumer culture is seen to reward self-indulgence, self-gratification or pleasure seeking. On the other hand, within consumer culture, the body shaped by the corporeal specificity of drug consumption is not proclaimed as a vehicle of pleasure. While, as we saw earlier, the drug-consuming female body is both a creation and a material resource, this female body is constructed by a variety of disciplinary regimes, although outflows from everyday hegemonic discourses happen. And these outflows will determine how these female bodies are rewarded in the drug consumption culture and whether or not these bodies can be vehicles of pleasure.

Drug-consuming bodies and consumption themes

In the book *Consumption and everyday life*, Hugh MacKay (1997) and his colleagues look at consumption using a wide-angled lens. In my view, their approach is useful in that their particular sociological focus is on consumption practices and everyday life. While the authors deal with a variety of forms of consumption as diverse as the print media, London shopping, TV soap operas, music, stories of place, broadcasting and information and communication technologies, they draw upon a series of key themes (what I refer to in this context as 'consumption themes') which include the balance between creativity and restraint; the interrelationship between consumption and production; the situated character of everyday practices; the broad range of consumption practices and the spatial dimension of consumption (MacKay, 1997: 11). As in previous discussions, I want to look at each theme and make links with drugs, gender and the body.

Creativity versus restraint

In his introduction, Hugh MacKay (1997: 11) notes that in examining the balance between creativity and constraint in consumption, we must place our analyses in everyday, local customs and practices. As we approach our analyses of consumption, he wants us to envisage imaginative, energetic persons working with an array of materials and through a series of consumption practices, creating and making sense of everyday life (MacKay, 1997: 11).

With special reference to drug consumption, we have, on the one hand, a meaning of the self as 'storied', the consuming drug user's 'self-narratives' as a medium through which she/he plays a creative role in formulating both her/his own identities, and the consumer culture in which she/he participates (Finnegan, 1997: 77). On the other hand, we have particular consumption processes and practices which are exclusionary or hegemonic and within which narratives of the self may get distorted or even lost (Thrift, 1997). Although there is a wide range of possible drug-consumption behaviours, given the many cultural sites and situations for drug consumption, the self-narratives of drug-consuming bodies are indeed constrained by the very fact that their cultural and moral disruptiveness is somehow embodied and therefore marked in some way (Urla and Terry, 1995). Nevertheless narratives of drug users, particularly women drug users, can evidence a type of creative consumption in which tensions between the self-expression and pleasure nexus become somehow resolved (Hinchliff, 2001).

Consumption and production

With regard to the next consumption theme, the interrelationship between consumption and production, Mackay (1997: 11) contends that, given the active nature of consumption and the fact that production is informed by the creative work of consumption in everyday life, consumption can be seen as a productive activity. In this way, the distinction between both conceptions, consumption and production, can be collapsed.

Celia Lury (1996: 123) describes this subsiding of the distinction between consumption and production in terms of the importance of recognizing circuits or cycles of production and consumption within society as a whole. Specifically, with regard to drug users, using drugs may be an instant of consumption but in the work of selecting, transporting and packaging the resources of drug consumption – drug supplies – these practices can also be seen as drug production. Additionally, women drug users can be actively involved in these circuits of production and consumption (Anderson, 2005; Hutton, 2005; Denton and O'Malley, 1999), as we have seen.

In this context, Fagan's (1995) female consumers and producers had distinct careerist concerns and were able to gather some cultural power in rapidly changing social structures in urban centres. Here we must not lose sight of how the embodied deviance of drug consumption and production is a fundamental feature of drug economies and markets. More importantly, we must keep in our minds the fact that racialization and gendering processes will also shape how these circuits, economies and markets become visible within restrictive and well-bounded social structures and how these operate in a male hegemonic way.

Situatedness

In looking at the situated character of everyday consumption practices, Mackay (1997: 11) directs us to the contexts of consumption and how things are appropriated and transformed by use in everyday life. At this point, his focus is on the relationship between the public and private or the outside world and private sphere and the mediation of the boundaries between them. We saw in an earlier discussion in this chapter how, as drug-consuming bodies offer themselves up to public consumption and are assessed on the adequacy of their performance of selves, this implies a mediation of the boundaries between the public and the private.

Perhaps it is easier to see how these boundaries can be mediated when we look beyond drug consumption to the consumption and production of information and communication technologies or when we recognize that place and identity are caught up in new forms of publicness (Thrift, 1997: 187). For example, we have new forms of mediated experiences when through circuits of consumption and production we have a connection to people in distinct parts of an interconnected world where key earth-shattering events are taking place.

Conceivably it is easier for us to envisage the mediation of the boundaries between the public and the private in other areas of consumption than drug consumption. It is true that in drug consumption contexts, illegal drugs as products are not advertized on billboards, on TV, on radio, and so on. Nevertheless a mediation of these boundaries does exist when, for example, as we saw earlier, drug users organize politically as veritable consumers and demand their human rights. It also happens when pregnant female bodies reject wholeheartedly the punitive familial ideology (Boyd, 1999) which determines the state's response to their stigmatized drug consumption.

Hugh MacKay (1997: 4) argues that our identity is made up by our consumption of goods: consumption and display constitute our expression of taste. Significantly, all of us have a series of embodied identities which may reflect both normativities and deviance. We may have a variety of consumption and production identities and, interestingly enough, drug user may be just one of these identities.

Range of consumer practices

Unlike Lury and Featherstone, Mackay (1997) and his colleagues do not attempt to link postmodernism and consumer society. Furthermore, Mackay (1997: 11) contends that their 'pleasure of consumption' approach conflates the two concepts. Regardless of whether of not his is a 'correct' analysis, Mackay wants to focus on what he calls a broad range of consumption practices and avoid analyses of stylized consumption, displays of consumption or at least shopping.

For our immediate purposes I am not so much interested in the range of consumption practices, given that in comparison to practices in general consumption, practices in the world of drug consumption may appear to be limited. Nevertheless I want to relate this idea of range of consumer practices specifically to drug-consuming bodies. Here I am drawn to the work of Frank (1995: 45–6) who analyses what he refers to as the mirroring body which defines itself in acts of consumption. For example, Frank sees that it is through consumption that the body becomes the instrument and object of consumption and aims to recreate itself in the image of others in style and health – the mirror image comes through here.

We saw previously that the drug-consuming body contradicts images of public health. Nevertheless this image of the mirroring body is able to exist for illegal drug consumers. In particular consuming drugs for female users has been aestheticized. This is in the sense that the standards by which drug consumption is judged have come to include not only prohibitive standards of pollution, contamination, and so on, but also a range of practices which appear in popular culture as style, glamour and chic. This is in light of the fact that globally known supermodels like Kate Moss and Naomi Campbell are seen to consume these forbidden products. Here female beauty can be seen to mix with drugs and social squalor, as model-ling designer clothes is included in the range of drug-consumption practice, targeting women. Here the female drug-using body becomes a bona fide mirroring body and the instrument and object of cultural consumption.

Consumption space

Mackay (1997: 11) highlights the spatial dimension of consumption and the fact that consumption takes place in space. He contends that consumption shapes spatial patterning of consumers and binds places together. In his view, we can now speak of local articulation of global processes. In an earlier discussion in this chapter, I spoke of an increase in sites for drug purchase and drug consumption and we saw that democratization of the contexts in which drugs are bought and sold have not included women.

Over and above these contexts, we are able to speak of the global drug economy and global drug markets (Gray, 1998) in the world of drug consumption. The key point here is that while an injecting pros-titute in London and a female crack dealer in New York may appear to have nothing in common except the fact that they are consuming drugs, they are perhaps able to share in new kinds of imagined communities with their own powers over place and space (Thrift, 1997). This is all about a progressive sense of place in which old forms of social exclusion and hegemonic power give way to a transnational sense of identity, place and space. In the end, drug users can effect work of cultural redefinition and require new stories about places and identities of themselves. Drug-consuming bodies need to learn to be both in and out of mainstream culture. We have certainly seen that, particularly for drug-consuming offenders, a programme like Project Worth in the USA (Welle, Falkin and Jainchill, 1998) appears to serve women, allowing them to address their victimization exper-iences as an integral, if not central feature of women's illegal drug consumption in a normative, perhaps global setting. In conclusion, the aim of this chapter has been to demonstrate within a sociology of consumption perspective how gendered drug users become visible in culturally specific ways and how they attain social and individual affirmation through drug consumption. While drug users, and in particular female drug users, live on the margins of society and experience a certain amount of prejudice and cultural gagging, they are key participants in a drug-consuming culture. This is true even though these women may be limited in their engagement with drug-consumption politics. The key point here is that looking at women drug users through the lens of consumption allows us to see more clearly how consumption issues affect women drug users' embodiment differently from men drug users'. Whether or not both groups see themselves as drug consumers, women's embodied consuming is certainly constructed as more stigmatizing than men's and morally more constraining. Yes, the mirroring body may define itself in acts of consumption, but the bodies of women drug users more than men drug users will need to be more vigilant as they recreate themselves in the image of others in style and health. This is especially true if these mirroring bodies are pregnant bodies, as we shall see in the next chapter.

6
Drug-Using Reproducing Bodies

> Patriarchal childbirth – childbirth as penance and as medical emergency – and its sequel, institutionalized motherhood, is alienated labor, exploited labor, keyed to an 'efficiency' and a profit system having little to do with the needs of mothers and children, carried on in physical and mental circumstances over which the woman in labor has little or no control. It is exploited labor in a form even more devastating than that of the enslaved industrial worker who has at least no psychic and physical bond with the sweated product, or with the bosses who control her. Not only have conception, pregnancy and birth been expropriated from women, but also the deep paraphysical sensations and impulses with which they are saturated.
>
> Adrienne Rich (1977: 163)

Inscribing chaos on pregnant drug-using bodies

Hopefully, readers will have a developing sense that over the past decades, indeed centuries, scientific and biomedical discourses on the body have become rooted in contemporary culture. As social scientists begin to position bodies centrally in their approaches to society and culture (E. Martin, 1992; Turner, 1996; Frank, 1995; Shilling, 2005; Featherstone, 1982; Davis, 1997; Bordo, 1993a; 1993b), natural scientists and biomedical experts persist with creating techniques to alter the boundaries of these bodies and attempt to close up the spaces between them. Often this has meant that social issues are not only allowed but also forced to emigrate to our bodies. Perhaps you the reader are beginning to see that the at times troubling social and cultural issue of drug use is emigrating in this way. In effect, we have all unwittingly become members of a captive audience to the cultural spectacle of drug use. Of course for drug-using women this spectacle has damaging consequences.

In this chapter, we turn our attention to another type of embodiment that is on offer to drug-using women, the reproducing body. Here I will draw attention to the regulatory regime or institution of reproduction in which a variety of powerful disciplinary practices determine what sorts of bodies should be reproductive and, of course, pregnant 'addicts' are 'off the radar' in this respect. At this juncture I aim to trace the cultural representations of pregnancy and drug use with regard to our 'body obsessed' society, examine the regulatory regime of reproduction with special reference to pregnancy and drugs and look closely at the 'real' material sites or gendered bodies upon which the chaos and disorder of drug use are inscribed.

Given this aim I will discuss four interrelated issues related to drug-using reproducing bodies. Firstly, I want to look at reproductive bodies, both drug-using and non-drug-using, within what we can refer to as the somatic society. Secondly, I want to look at how 'normal' or 'deviant' and non-drug-using or drug-using pregnant bodies become visible and indeed visualized through the 'scopic drive', a characteristic of this somatic society. Thirdly, related to the somatic society with its scopic drive is the regulatory regime of reproduction which I want to explore with regard to its disciplinary practices directed towards drug-using pregnant bodies. Lastly, I present and analyse my ideas on women, drugs and pregnancy and look specifically at pregnant drug-using bodies as 'material sites' related to the notion of 'disordered body'. Here the idea of resistance to the dominant ideology of reproduction emerges.

The assumption which underlies the development of ideas in this chapter is that the pregnant drug-using body is constructed as a deviant body, a discursive construct which is separated from other female bodies and deciphered by experts as being immoral, inferior, disgusting and 'out of order'. This process generates a controlling response and has devastating intended and unintended consequences for these gendered, drug-using bodies.

Reproductive bodies and drugs in the somatic society

Reproduction is an important aspect of social and cultural corporeality in the somatic society which is defined by Bryan Turner (1992: 12–13) 'as a social system in which the body, as simultaneously constraint and resistance, is the principal field of cultural and political activity – a system which is structured around regulating bodies'. For Turner, the body in the somatic society becomes the dominant means by which the crisis and tensions of society are thematized. The body makes available the material for our political ruminations as we learn that our cultures are obsessed with bodies.

For example, experts frequently ask the questions: How do bodies move? What do bodies consume? How do bodies get sick? How do bodies stay healthy? What do bodies look like? How do bodies differ from the 'norm'? What is the body 'norm'? What colours or race are bodies? How do bodies appear? When?, How? and With whom do bodies have sex or not have sex? How old or young are bodies? How do bodies change? What do bodies ingest? Do bodies decorate or mark themselves? How do bodies die? These sorts of questions are asked in the somatic society with one overriding aim: to regulate and control bodies. In this way, the clout of staking cultural and political ruminations and claims through the body rests on the assumption that bodies, like property, are real material objects whose dispositions are of great concern to society as a whole (Urla and Terry, 1995: 6). The feminist adage 'the personal is political' may still ring true today. The fact that material, gendered bodies continue to be political targets merely helps us to extend our feminist ontological and political concerns to more cultures of resistance.

In the somatic society, women's bodies, and specifically their prenatal, reproductive spaces or wombs, became construed over time as the battlefield for the social body's survival (Stormer, 2000: 118). These reproductive bodies become the substance of our ideological reflections on human life in a world of risk, insecurity and disorder. In the nineteenth century, women's reproductive organs began to coincide with colonial nation states' perception that their material landscapes were apparently lacking sufficient White populations (Stormer, 2000: 118). Today, the White majority's heterosexual, able-bodied, young, female wombs perform a functional role by normalizing prenatal space in a society obsessed with regulating reproductive bodies. In the contemporary drugs field, when poor, pregnant, African-American women produce 'crack babies' (Humphries, 1999) or 'infant addicts', these deviant bodies are able to connect institutionalized racism and sexism to biological reproduction, while being increasingly targeted and oppressed in the battleground of the social body's 'war against drugs'.

The biopolitics and concerns of somatic society revolve around controlling reproduction (rather than increasing production) and regulating the spaces between bodies – to monitor the interfaces between bodies, societies and culture as well as to legislate the tensions between habitus (that is, life world of actors or cultural codes) and the body (Turner, 1992: 12). Bryan Turner contends that we want to close up bodies by promoting safe sex, using clean needles, and so on. In this context, the pregnant drug user becomes a visible feature, if not potent symbol of the somatic society. She exposes how the personal and public problem of 'drug addiction' during pregnancy can reflect simultaneously embodied desires for an unfettered womb and an open ingesting body, as well as the cultural need for bodily restriction, control and regulation. Of course, her race, class and age will govern both the formulation of her desires and the way culture controls these seemingly 'uncontrollable' desires.

In the somatic society, treating women as mere uterine environments that can be invaded or punished involves the kind of blaming-the-victim mentality that can only seem proper when one completely ignores the complex social conditions surrounding prenatal harm to future persons (Callahan and Knight, 1992: 235). Blaming pregnant drug users is all about wanting to close up these 'deviant' female bodies and regulate them physically and psychologically, while at the same time denying that self-surveillance within the context of a desire for a positive fetal outcome (Irwin, 1995) may exist for many, if not all of these women.

From a feminist point of view, a series of significant suspicions can be raised in this context, given that the disciplinary power of the drug treatment system often operates to adjust these pregnant drug-using women to dominant gender, race and class structures, as well as depoliticizes and individualizes their situations (Young, 1994: 33–34). One can rightly ask, Who really benefits from this type of drug treatment system? Surely, it is not pregnant women. Related to this issue of benefiting from treatment, previous research

(Pursley-Crotteau and Stern, 1996) has shown that pregnant women in treatment who are going through the developmental process of achieving a 'maternal identity' found that their psychological and biological needs often conflicted with the treatment philosophy that was offered to them.

As implied from the discussions above, the ideal body in the somatic society is a conforming body, not a deviant one. Thus, a drug-using body, particularly a female pregnant one, falls short of this conforming body ideal. In general the pregnant body is constructed both as a docile subject, submitting to invasive medical scrutiny, and as an active agent, responsible for optimizing fetal health (Lee and Jackson, 2002: 126). On the other hand, for the pregnant drug-using body her docility and active agency appear as questionable, if not vigorously denied by society. This denial may be one reason why attempts are made in the drug treatment system to give pregnant drug users treatment priority (Arfken et al, 2002; Carter, 2002; Curet and Hsi, 2002; Nishimoto and Roberts, 2001; Greberman and Jasinski, 2001; Rosenbaum and Irwin, 2000): these women are constructed as being wild, out of control bodies. This cultural denial of these women's agency and normality implies that their bodies, as well as their fetuses are worthless.

Ironically in the somatic society, bodies become more conforming, compliant or obedient when they become healthier and less ill, as well as more ill and less healthy. Either way, they are drawn into some form of self and cultural governance. Both conceptions, health and illness, are culturally and socially constructed and all cultures have known disciplinary practices and regulatory regimes surrounding the notions of health and illness. That the notions of health and illness can be embodied, and furthermore are able to be translated into notions of 'good' or 'bad' and 'normal' or 'deviant' bodies, reflects the fact that morality is deeply embedded in the discourses of health, wellbeing and disease. Of course, a similar process is visible with regard to the discourse of drug use, as drug-using bodies are constructed as 'bad'/'deviant' bodies. Drug users are perceived as socially, physically and mentally diseased individuals. Given that the somatic society is concerned with regulating reproductive bodies as a fundamental activity of social, cultural and political life, women's drug-using bodies are centrally located and become visible or represented as 'bad'/ 'deviant'/'diseased' bodies in need of regulation, restraint and control.

Becoming visible: visualization through the scopic drive

As implied above, the disciplinary practices and regulatory regimes surrounding health and illness in the somatic society can be seen to mirror those surrounding the drugs discourse. These practices and regimes vary from culture to culture according to how ill or healthy, 'good' or 'bad' and 'normal' or 'deviant' bodies become visible and, as we shall see, are visualized. Importantly, these practices and regimes differ according to the extent and range of the scopic drive (Braidotti, 1994: 64) in science and medicine. The scopic drive is a powerful cultural force which categorizes 'normal' or 'deviant' bodies and achieves biomedical aims by making embodied subjects observable and comprehensible according to the ideology of scientific representation.

Here it is interesting to consider what addiction specialists refer to as the molecular basis of addiction (de Belleroche, 2002) when pleasure centres and reinforcement centres in neurons, as well as adaptive responses to cell signalling are visualized. These scientific representations disembody the drug user (for example, her body is absent), while at the same time exposing how troublesome addictions can be represented visually on a cellular level. This unique process involves the commodification of the scopic and the triumph of vision over the other senses (Braidotti, 2002: 246). In effect for the biomedical expert, seeing is believing. Rosi Braidotti (2002: 246) is concerned with this vision-centred approach to thought, knowledge and science, characterized by this scopic drive which turns visualization into a crucial form of governance. This invincible, scopic drive not only breaks the connection between seeing and the mind but also denies embodiment by visualizing what's in bodies through seeing technologies or strategies such as ultrasound, MRI scanners, high-powered microscopes, or more traditional pictorial representations of cellular processes.

In our era, we are experiencing the omnipresence of the visual – visualization has been turned into the ultimate form of control. The triumph of this scopic drive, or what I call disembodied vision, is that it is a clear gesture of science's epistemological domination and control to make visible the invisible and to visualize the secrets of nature (Braidotti, 1994: 64). Pregnant bodies may be the objects of medical scrutiny and surveillance as what is in their wombs becomes more visible, but these bodies are also sources of discomfort and disgust in popular culture (Stabile, 1994: 84).

Furthermore it is difficult to conceptualize pregnant embodiment given that there are striking taboos surrounding representations of the pregnant body in visual culture (Tyler, 2001: 74). Nevertheless visualization can be an important means of controlling pregnant drug users in a variety of settings – on the street dealing or buying, with her partner, at home, in work, in treatment, in prison, and so on. If and when her pregnancy is visible, she is likely to be more vulnerable to the vagaries of her social situation.

While cultural representations of pregnant women depict this body as vulnerable and in need of protection, by using drugs, pregnant women are perceived as consciously abandoning that sort of protection and putting their bodies and fetuses in jeopardy. The pregnant drug user is the embodiment of risk. A pregnant drug user is viewed as doubly disgusting – she is pregnant and she consumes drugs. In this context, whether sick or healthy, drug-using or non-drug-using' 'good' or 'bad', male, female, transgendered or intersexed, Black, brown, White or coloured, and so on bodies scrutinized by the scopic drive are inevitably merely experimental objects. Here there is an assumed transparency of bodies. For pregnant drug users, this assumed transparency means that 'seeing' into her womb or visualizing her embodiment reveals not only fetal but also social damage.

Side by side with the scopic drive generated by science and medicine is a powerful desire to classify all forms of deviance, situate them in biology and guard them in wider cultural and social spaces. Key embodiment theorists Jacqueline Urla and Jennifer Terry (1995:1) contend that since the nineteenth century the somatic territorializing of deviance has been part and parcel of a larger effort to organize social relations according to categories denoting health versus pathology, normality versus abnormality and national security versus social danger. Moreover for these theorists (Urla and Terry, 1995: 2), deviance, translated into the early twenty-first century, has become a matter of somatic essence facilitated by moral discourses surrounding addiction and other anomalies of bodies. They argue that as a result of these complex culturally embodied processes, bodies have become marked and social relations organized in terms of deviant and conforming bodies. Crucially, pressing social issues and cultural concerns are being displaced onto the body.

However, before cultural conceptions of normal or abnormal, conformity or non-conformity and health or pathology can be formed, there needs to exist a collection of bodies upon which these categories can be inscribed. In particular, the unique process of inscribing bodies as 'healthy' or 'diseased', 'good' or 'bad', 'ordered' or 'disordered' and 'lovely' or 'monstrous', and so on, is performed by authoritative discourses and scientific practices, targeting bodies. In the drugs field, a whole series of discourses and practices shape the drug-using body as somatically different from the non-drug-using body. When a fetus is added to this equation, the moral character of the pregnant female body is put into question. She is viewed not only as behaviourally aberrant but also as socially disruptive by the very fact that she uses drugs while pregnant. As we have seen, she embodies disgust both by being pregnant and by consuming illegal drugs. More importantly, the cultural fear is that by embodying disgust she will reproduce something disgusting – a fetus – which will be ghastly, deformed or less than normal.

Mixing drugs with the regulatory regime of reproduction

As we saw in Chapter 2, all bodies must confront the bodily task of reproduction upon which society sets certain cultural requirements. In this context, Bryan Turner (1996: 109) contends that for every society there is a strict disciplinary regime and bodily order which means that society is compelled to reproduce its members. The discipline of Western, urbanized civilization with its neo-liberal ideology is one requiring that most, if not all citizens reproduce.

In terms of procreation and replicating bodies, medical and other experts' disembodied visions of these bodies have had a major impact on contemporary notions of reproduction. Consistently, the future embodied products of these procreative gendered bodies have taken priority over the process of reproduction (Newman, 1996). In this context, I would contend that, similar to gender (Lorber, 1994), reproduction as a component of culture is exhibiting signs of a social institution. It is becoming visible as a distinct regulatory regime.

As reproduction ascends in this way, it matures into a regulatory regime focused on the making of bodies which should embody wholeness (that is, limbs, torsos, crania filled with brains, and so on), health, wellbeing and society's future welfare. Thus reproduction appears as a multifarious organization of activities and social relations, embodying notions of able-bodiness, heterosexuality, human survival, progress, citizenship and being drug free! At the same time, reproductive bodies, both drug-using and non-drug-using, become more valorized than ever before through scientific and medical discourses.

Thus as a normative system reproduction controls the actions of procreative bodies – both male bodies and female bodies. But given that female more than male bodies are seen as reproductive, the procreative bodies of females are subject to more control than those of males. Indeed, there is a multiplicity of practices and disciplines guiding pregnant bodies as these bodies are marshalled together in a systematic way under the banner of reproduction. The symbol of the emergent regulatory regime of reproduction is the pregnant body, the body of a woman producing a newborn, as well as the chemicals, hormones, eggs, cells, genes, blood, fetal tissues – all gathered, drawn, scraped, tested, examined, and at times discarded within the regulatory regime of reproduction (see also Ettorre, 2002: 2–5, for a discussion of the institution of reproduction vis-à-vis contemporary genetics). A variety of disciplinary strategies (that is, technologies of the self, biotechnologies, discourses, and so on) attend to the pregnant body to construct and normalize this body, while regulatory techniques are played out through science, law and medicine. Of course, if these pregnant bodies are viewed as deviant ones, such as pregnant drug users, these normalizing strategies gather cultural momentum.

While drug use in pregnancy holds the interest of clinicians and public health officials alike (Markovic et al., 2000), this type of drug use tends to produce a punishment response (Young, 1994), as well as scapegoating policies which are not conducive to the wellbeing of the pregnant user (Paone and Alpern, 1998). In this area moral panics are often generated relating to society's perceptions regarding the race, class (Duster, 1970: 20–1) and gender of those who are using drugs. It is a shame that empathy is lacking in these cultural responses, as previous research (Fiorentine, Nakashima and

Anglin, 1999) suggests that women drug users, particularly those in treatment, respond favourably to an empathic environment.

In order to best contextualize the notion of embodiment and to understand the conditions and experiences of embodiment vis-à-vis living, reproducing, female drug-using bodies, we need to be cognisant of a whole series of complex cultural practices and moral discourses which target these pregnant bodies. If we return to the ideas of Rosi Braidotti (1994: 80), we see that within a logocentric economy and phallocentric discursive order there is a traditional association of women with monstrosity. In this context Braidotti uses the image of a pregnant body to provide clarity. For example, a woman's body can change shape in pregnancy and childbearing. The pregnant body defies the notion of fixed bodily form – visible, recognisable, clear and distinct shape as that which marks the contours of the body (Braidotti, 1994: 80). What's more, the pregnant body is 'morphologically dubious'; the fact that this female body can change shape so drastically is 'troublesome' within the context of the logocentric economy within which to see (as we saw earlier) is the primary act of knowledge (Braidotti, 1994: 80).

On a similar ontological level, Longhurst (2001: 81) contends that pregnant embodiment disrupts dualistic thinking, given that expectant women go through a bodily process that transgresses the boundaries between inside and outside, self and other, one and two, mother and fetus, subject and object. Furthermore when occupying public space pregnant bodies are to be dreaded not trusted, given that they threaten to break their boundaries, to spill or to leak (Longhurst, 2001: 82). When drugs are placed within this cultural mix, pregnant drug users not only upset dualistic thinking but also represent leaky bodies who endow dangerous substances with mystical properties (Sedgwick, 1994: 132). Taking these magical or mind-altering supplements (that is, drugs) is seen to operate corrosively on the self and thus imply a lack of moral fibre. The pregnant drug-using body is not only the abject or monstrous body who threatens to leak but also the 'bad' body whose leakiness contaminates the rational, public world of the logocentric economy. This body infects or contaminates the intimate, private spaces related to inside and outside, self and other and mother and fetus.

If we look at the social and cultural processes marking the boundaries between 'good' and 'bad' bodies, we see some of

the cultural components of the scientific, legal and medical ortho-
doxies which shape these reproductive female bodies as abnormal
bodies. Within the regulatory regime of reproduction we need to
envisage the reproductive body and, more specifically, the drug-
using, reproductive body as the end-product of a whole system of
cultural relations.

Drug use in pregnancy is heavily stigmatized and can be legally
punishable (Goldstein et al, 2000: 356). Indeed, coercive and punitive
sanctions can be imposed on pregnant or post-pregnant female
bodies. These measures may include: incarceration to prevent damage
or further damage to a fetus or invoking criminal sanctions such as
being charged with reckless homicide; criminal mistreatment of a
child; reckless endangerment, child abuse and child neglect (Deville
and Kopeland, 1998: 239–40). While pointing out that many women
will be punished for behaviour that results in no harm to the
newborn, these authors (Deville and Kopeland, 1998: 251) rightly
ask, 'In what other context does society punish individuals crimin-
ally with potential imprisonment merely for creating a risk of harm?'
Furthermore, to get pregnant women into treatment other criminal
and civil approaches may involve treatment in lieu of prosecution,
involuntary civil commitment, removing child custody and denial of
public benefits (Nishimoto and Roberts, 2001: 162).

These types of harsh disciplinary practices are not just about the
surveillance of pregnant bodies within the institution of reproduction. They are also about the cultural imperative impelling women to
perform 'correctly' or 'normatively' with their pregnant bodies in the
regulatory regime of reproduction. We know that one basic requirement of this regime is that reproducers, especially female ones, should
be free from any and all substances viewed as harmful, addictive or
mind altering. This requirement is linked to the cultural expectation
which is part of a more general, fairly recent trend towards increasingly severe 'rules of pregnancy' (Oaks, 2001: 19). These new 'rules
of pregnancy' are derived from the medical professions' changing
knowledge on fetal health and furthermore result in a visible biomedical policing of pregnant women's lifestyles (Paone and Alpern,
1998).

While Laury Oaks (2001) looks specifically at pregnancy through
the lens of women smokers, we are able to recognize similar 'rules of
pregnancy' or stringent disciplinary practices operating for women

drug users. For example, Oaks (2001: 19) contends that the discovery over the years that women's reproductive biology (read bodies) fails to protect the fetus has strengthened the idea that women's behaviour while pregnant must be regulated and supervized by health professionals, as well as by each pregnant woman herself. But of course the 'pregnant addict' is viewed as incapable of regulating her own health and behaviour. For her, 'rules of pregnancy' usually mean the experience of stigma and discrimination in relation not only to her drug use but also to her race, gender and socioeconomic status (Abercrombie and Booth, 1997).

In this context all pregnant bodies are directed by physicians and scientific experts to play out their reproductive roles in biomedically approved ways, as these bodies are pushed into the service of 'doing pregnancy' the correct way. The fact that a pregnant woman is a subject situated within a labouring body with her own point of view (Sbisa, 1996) tends to be minimized by clinicians within the institution of reproduction. Any woman's choice to take drugs is seen not only to pollute her reproducing body but also to be regarded by others as unnatural, deviant, selfish or evil (Lewis, 2002: 40).

Susan Bordo (1993a: 93) contends that in contemporary society women's reproductive rights are being fought over as well as their status as subjects within cultural arrangements in which, for better or worse, the safeguarding of the 'real' subject, the foetus, is central. In an attempt to understand why the cultural idiom of reproduction has such credible social power, we are able to see important, sometimes not so visible, social processes and disciplinary practices being played out. This is especially true when we attempt to envisage this cultural idiom through the lens of drug use. In this context, Sheigla Murphy and Marsha Rosenbaum (1999: 1) note that when people believe the hand that rocks the cradle would rather be taking drugs, various constituencies unite in moral outrage and condemnation – for women, drug use is viewed as the antithesis of responsible behaviour and good health during pregnancy.

Pregnancy, drugs and the disordered body

As implied in the above discussions, at its core the regulatory regime of reproduction privileges an individualistic, mechanistic view of the pregnant female body with the result that the full importance of the cultural and biological processes of reproduction is lost for many of these women. Of course this view, modelled on the workings of an inorganic object, is not new in medicine, science and culture. Within this sort of paradigm the body is ministered to as a machine and it is the doctor, the mechanic, who repairs it (E. Martin, 1992). It is interesting to note that conceptions formulated within 'the body as machine' perspective facilitate the maintenance of gender prejudices rather than gender impartiality (Mahowald, 1994). Indeed, the science of biomedicine is embedded in gendered social practices and like all gendered social practices (Lorber, 1997: 3), these are able to transform bodies.

While drug use may alter the bodies of those who use drugs (see de Belleroche, 2002), pregnant drug users are affected in particular by scientific research on reproduction and childbirth in which gendered practices and norms are embedded. Scientific research helps to establish, manage and perpetuate the 'rules of pregnancy' which affect all pregnant women, drug using or not. Joan Bertin (1995: 384) contends that certain tendencies are entrenched in this type of scientific research and these include an overstatement of women's biological and behavioural responsibility for the wellbeing of the next generation; an underestimation of the importance of paternal biological and behavioural factors for the wellbeing of the next generation; and the use of scientific maxims to reinforce social behavioural norms, particularly the definition of appropriate behaviour.

Pregnant drug users feel the brunt of these tendencies and usually experience an acute sense of how 'bad' they 'do pregnancy'. While women drug users are generally pathologized (Haller, Miles and Dawson, 2002; Jainchill, Hawke and Yagelka, 2000) and viewed as scientifically disordered, pregnant drug users tend to become the objects of disgust in contemporary culture. Disgust is seen to take over these material sites (for example, pregnant drug-using bodies) as 'objects'. Disgust is a type of all-encompassing affective embodiment. Disgust is the very designation of badness that society assumes is inherent in these bodies (Ahmed, 2004: 84).

Here scientific research and social disgust fuel the cultural and at times self-imposition of badness or at least guilt (Murphy and Rosenbaum, 1999: 69) for these drug-using women. Furthermore, if and when these women give birth and their drug use is extended to motherhood, some researchers believe that their irresponsible, embodied choices reflect 'the chaotic values of the mother's behaviour regarding the needs of the child' (Stocco, Calafat and Mendes, 2000: 15). In the end, a pregnant drug user is viewed as being in a no-win situation bodily, emotionally, relationally and culturally.

Linking the pregnant drug-using body to the discourse of scientific research I want to look briefly at Susan Bordo's (1993a) critique of biomedicine in an attempt to further elucidate disordered embodiment. She (Bordo, 1993a: 67) contends that the body of the subject in the medical model is the passive tablet on which 'disorder' is inscribed and deciphering that inscription is the working domain of the medical expert who alone can unlock the secrets of this disordered body. These notions suggest that the injunction on activity and focus on disorder may have special effects on pregnant women who experience all sorts of gendering practices when masculinist science re-conceptualizes reproduction as a technological rather than natural process.

Within the regulatory regime of reproduction, governed by these scientists and biomedical experts, pregnant women are encouraged to treat their bodies as passive instruments of new emergent technologies (Bordo, 1993a: 86). For pregnant drug users it would be disastrous if they treated their bodies as 'passive instruments'. As pregnant users they need, in order to survive and 'do a successful pregnancy', a type of active embodiment which may involve choosing strategies for reducing drug-related harm such as switching to 'safer' drugs; counteracting drug use by taking vitamins and other remedies; altering their drug-using lifestyles by forcing themselves to sleep or moving from drug-using neighbourhoods and, in some instances, seeking prenatal care (Rosenbaum and Irwin, 2000).

Regardless of these survival strategies for pregnant drug users, recent developments in biomedicine shape new values for the standards of reproduction – values to which all pregnant women, even pregnant drug users, are told they must conform. In this context, for the feminist theorist the disordered body, like all gendered bodies, is engaged in a process of making meaning, of 'labour on the body' (Bordo, 1993a: 67). Here the notion of reproduction as a valuable material site of embodied experience for all women emerges. Nonetheless we must work hard and labour so that feminine ontology of the female body is privileged, especially when we are looking at a specific form of reproductive embodiment that presents opportunities for resistance, for making meanings that oppose or evade the dominant ideology (Bordo, 1993b: 193).

From this feminist standpoint, drug use during pregnancy is under no circumstances purely selfish, self-indulgent, irresponsible or bad, under no circumstances purely a fall from grace or embodiment of evil. Nor is being pregnant while using drugs facilitated by cultural images of 'crack whores' or 'pregnant addicts'. Drug use during pregnancy is not 'behaviour derived from immorality rather than from illness' (Paone and Alpern, 1998: 101) nor a license for doctors to treat pregnant users harshly (Boyd, 1999: 66). Rather drug use during pregnancy may be an attempt to embody particular cultural values and norms and to construct a gendered, expectant body that will speak for itself in a consequential and powerful way. For example, these pregnant drug users may use drugs to cope with the strains of family life (Raine, 2001) or to increase their sense of authority or control over their difficult situations (Taylor, 1993). For pregnant women, drugs can be used as a resource or a survival strategy to help them endure the problems they face as women drug users and victims of abuse (Sales and Murphy, 2000: 709) or to make their lives more manageable and inclusive of at least some leisure.

Paloma Sales and Sheigla Murphy's (2000) research in this area revealed that drugs were used by pregnant women to relieve pain, to create a sense of control or to prevent partner violence and abuse. Other research demonstrated that worries or fears about the welfare of others were important for these women, especially their concerns for the welfare of their children (Copeland, 1998: 333; Baker and Carson, 1999). Obviously, the cultural belief that presumes these pregnant women are uncaring and totally irresponsible is erroneous.

Women drug users are not merely 'victims' of their circumstances but by using drugs may be attempting to cope with a range of issues in their lives in which drug use forms part of a coping strategy (Malloch, 2004: 388). Nevertheless in order to manage their status as pregnant drug users, women need to navigate a safe passage through a series of perceived risks, such as losing custody of their children, causing fetal damage or being severely stigmatized in public settings (Irwin, 1995: 635). Here pregnant drug-using bodies are capable of being employed as a conduit for the expression of a variety of at times conflicting concerns, desires and predicaments, existing in society.

Within this type of viewpoint, illuminating drug use in pregnancy does not necessitate expert knowledge. Rather what is needed is attentiveness to the myriad strata of cultural representations that are embedded in this type of gendered, 'disordered body'.

For example, ideas surrounding pregnancy in contemporary society are spurred on by the surveillance practices of biomedical experts and materialize as resistance to autonomous motherhood (De Gama, 1993). Furthermore beneath the compelling cultural apprehension of drug-addicted babies and the development of public health programmes designed for the special needs of certain populations, especially minority women, who are or would like to be pregnant (Balsamo, 1999: 241) lies a basic animosity and resistance to women's self-governance (Campbell, 1999: 917).

This cultural animosity reveals the problematic and politicized nature of human reproduction and the fact that whether pregnant drug users bring their babies to term or have an abortion, they are unable to experience any form of normality in and through the biomedical discourse. Inevitably, as we saw in Chapter 3, female drug users will bear the three stigmata of being immoral, sexually indiscrete and inadequate caregivers – stigmata which become even more punitive when women are seen to abuse drugs during pregnancy and perpetuated by the unprofessional behaviour and pejorative attitudes of health care providers (Carter, 2002: 302).

It is important to note here that negative social responses to pregnant drug users, such as stigmatization and imputing legal liability, may impact disproportionately on racialized women and women of low economic status (Goldstein et al. 2000: 364–5). I believe there is a sense of urgency for treaters to be aware of the emotional, psychological, economic and social impacts of these issues and to try to actively engage *all women drug users* in caring environments (Curet and Hsi, 2002). The above type of negative expert response exists alongside controlled scientific reproduction (Spallone and Steinberg, 1987: 15) which not only fragments the meaning of motherhood (Hill Collins, 1999: 279) but also brings both the physician and the pregnant woman into a system of normative surveillance which for pregnant drug users means that the dominant narrative is one of maternal excess and fetal victimization (Balsamo, 1999: 243).

In conclusion, we have seen in this chapter that the cultural workings of reproduction, drugs and the gendered body expose the long-standing feminist unease that the medicalization of reproduction, pregnancy and childbirth has more often than not been against the interests of pregnant women, making them objects of medical care rather than subjects with agency and rational decision-making powers. Compound this situation with using drugs and we can rightly say that 'All hell breaks loose'. In the above discussions, I have outlined how cultural representations of pregnant drug users in the somatic society and within the regulatory regime of reproduction become 'eye food' for biomedical experts in their visualization of these disembodied female subjects. I have attempted to weave together the notions of pregnant drug use, somatic society, drug use, scopic drive, disgust and disordered bodies in order to demonstrate their symbolic relationship in popular culture.

As a feminist theorist I want to make meaning and labour on the drug-using reproducing body in order to further demonstrate how an embodiment approach is able to illuminate some of the complexities of pregnant drug users' intractable social situation. The very act of using drugs during pregnancy is confounding the dominant discourse on drugs and reproduction. For pregnant users there may be power and pleasure in this type of embodied cultural work. Resisting normalization may produce some benefits. At the very least their disordered bodies are resisting the grip of the regulatory regime of reproduction on their 'deviant' bodies and attempting to give those experts employing the all pervasive scopic drive a veritable black eye.

7
Contaminated Drug-Using Bodies

The Master-Maker in His making had made Old Death. Made Him with big, soft feet and square toes. Made him with a face that reflects the face of all things, but neither changes itself, nor is mirrored anywhere. Made the body of Death out of infinite hunger. Made a weapon for his hand to satisfy his needs. This was the morning of the day of the beginning of things. But Death had no home and he knew it at once. 'And where shall I dwell in my dwelling?' Old Death asked, for he was already old when he was made. 'You shall build a place close to the living, yet far out of the sight of eyes. Wherever there is a building, there you have a platform that comprehends the four roads of the winds. For your hunger, I give you the first and last taste of all things.' We had been born, so Death had his first taste of us. We had built things, so he had his platform in our yard. And now, Death stirred from his platform in his secret place in our yard, and came inside the house.

Zora Neale Hurston (1986: 27)

Offering a fresh approach

Since the beginning of the 'AIDS epidemic', prostitutes and injecting drug users have been blamed for transmitting HIV/AIDS to the heterosexual community. This emphasis on deviant bodies as cultural embodiments of material conduits of HIV/AIDS has been a consistent theme in public health policies and legal discourses, as well as biomedical and scientific research. Interestingly enough, it was the deviant bodies of female injecting drug users who accounted for the greatest number of reported cases of HIV/AIDS among Western women (Brook et al., 2000). While the impact on women's bodies on a global scale has been given some prominence in the HIV/AIDS debates, there are similarities between women at risk in places such as Africa and the United States – similarities which are socio-political, as well as rooted in poverty and power imbalances between the sexes (Wenzel and Tucker, 2005: 154).

Women's acquisition of the virus has grown more rapidly than men's. In 1998, drug use was seen to play a major role in the spread of this disease: 46 per cent of women's AIDS cases have been directly attributed to injecting drug use and another 18 per cent attributed to women's heterosexual contacts with injecting drug users (Coyle, 1998: 2). In 2002, women's AIDS cases directly attributed to injecting drug use grew to 62 per cent, while the percentage of cases attributed to women's heterosexual contacts with injecting drug users stabilized at 18 per cent (Bloom, 2002: 97). It appears that in comparison to male injecting drug users, it is more common for female injecting drug users to have a partner who is also an injecting drug user or one who is HIV positive (de la Hera et al., 2001).

Through the lens of feminist embodiment, I attempt in this chapter to contextualize HIV/AIDS as a disease that is not only changing human history (Barnett and Whiteside, 2002: 24) but also the drugs field. While this may be considered a grand claim, I think it is important to bear in mind how living with deadly 'dis-eases' such as drug use and HIV/AIDS brings up for us the issue of our humanity and what it means to be human in societies where experiencing pain, embodying dis-ease and confronting death have become moral issues, inscribed on our bodies.

At this point I want to emphasize the need for a fresh approach to the HIV/AIDS area where, in my view, the current one has become somewhat stale – its ideas rather worn-out. In the West the frenzied media panic of the 1980s, followed by the public health messages of the 1990s, have been replaced by a fake sense of security, based on widespread social denial and overt racism in the early twenty-first century. Given that Western countries share only five per cent of the global burden of 37 million HIV/AIDS cases worldwide (Barnett and Whiteside, 2002: 24; Ekanem and Gbadegesin, 2004), the false belief that HIV/AIDS is a treatable disease has emerged in the public's consciousness. Although this false belief may appear at first glance as bland it represents a dangerous type of denial. It aims towards the cultural maintenance of social worlds in which an undesirable condition such as HIV/AIDS is made to seem normal and this underlying theme of denial is integral to the story of HIV/AIDS (Cohen, 2001: 51, 56).

This type of normalization can result in a refusal to allocate resources to stigmatized groups, as well as obscure the impact of HIV/AIDS on people in Sub-Saharan Africa, Asia, Latin America, Eastern Europe and the former Soviet Union. An awareness of the growth of HIV/AIDS in these areas of the world can be used not only to preclude opportunities for economic growth but also as a basis for an extended medical surveillance of these disadvantaged populations (Turner, 1992: 11). Here we see that through cultural denial biomedicine is able to normalize bodies in the West while pathologizing those in 'the rest'. As a powerful strategy, normalization colours social and heath policy concerns which filter down to risk reduction schemes practiced amongst local communities perceived as being at risk, such as drug users. But the cultural denial involved in 'pretending' HIV/AIDS is a treatable disease may not apply as forcefully to drug users as other 'afflicted' groups. This is because drug users embody dirt, pollution and cultural immorality. We want death to take them off our hands. Drug users already embody depravity as a result of being embroiled (as we have seen earlier) in a much maligned 'epidemic of the will', drug addiction. Of course, women drug users embody even more degeneracy because their bodies should be 'purer' than men's.

In this chapter I attempt to establish a fresh approach to HIV/AIDS and injecting drug use and in doing this I want to flag up the importance of supporting an anti-oppressive discourse on HIV/AIDS. Given the above discussion, we should be able to sense that building up a fresh approach to HIV/AIDS and injecting drug use, while supporting an anti-oppressive, critical discourse, is perhaps timely. Of course, I want to develop and shape discussions in this chapter with a feminist-embodiment slant which I believe needs to be upheld and perpetuated. For me, to build up a new approach to HIV/AIDS and injecting drug users and to support a minority, anti-oppressive discourse is all about removing the obstacles or problems related to envisaging how the bodies of drug users, particularly women's, are constructed in terms of the categories laid out to them. I identify three problems which obscure this type of feminist embodiment and build discussions in this chapter around an elaboration of these problems. First, the usual focus around HIV/AIDS has been masculinist in its concerns, employing the male body as the standard against which HIV/AIDS is defined. Secondly, women's functionality vis-à-vis heterosexuality has been used destructively against women in the HIV/AIDS debate in which women's bodies are defined according to male heterosexual desire. Thirdly, the traditional linking of prostitution and drug use, or the existence of the 'whore, drugs and risk cultural configuration' in the drug misuse literature, has meant that a true picture of the experiences of female prostitutes, as well as of female drug users, is blurred. As I mentioned earlier I will structure this chapter according to discussions of these three problems. In the conclusion, I look critically at women drug users' bodies in what has been called the postmodern moment of HIV/AIDS.

The assumption which underlies the development of ideas in this chapter is that key structural, political and embodiment issues must be brought together in any discussion of HIV/AIDS. Our desire for social justice for those injecting drug users with HIV/AIDS who struggle for self-determination must be informed by the sense that we are constituted politically by virtue of the social vulnerability of our bodies (Butler, 2004: 18). An understanding of these issues and this desire is necessary for a comprehensive, cultural awareness of the impact of HIV/AIDS on female drug users' bodies.

In my recent review of research on women, HIV/AIDS and injecting drug use over a ten-year period from 1995 to 2005 (which, as mentioned earlier, I carried out in the course of writing this book), I noticed consistently that a full understanding of the complexities of these issues tends to be subverted, denied or indeed lost. In effect, when an appreciation of these issues is missing from relevant research and scientific frameworks, policies are implemented which reflect the allegation that drug use is a moral problem rather than a physical, psychological and social issue (Abercrombie and Booth, 1997: 182). Of course within these policy debates women suffer because they are branded as less than good or immoral, given that women continue to be perceived within popular culture as the custodians of morals. With these ideas in mind, I hope in this chapter to distinguish different discourses organizing the expression of the embodied experience of women injecting drug users confronting HIV/AIDS.

The traditional masculinist focus of concerns around HIV/AIDS

First, the HIV/AIDS issue has been defined in public health terms by employing white, Western, middle class, male bodies as the standard against which clinical HIV/AIDS is defined (Patton, 1990). Behind this defining process, or what Richardson (1996: 163) calls the male-ing of HIV/AIDS, is the male body representative of all bodies on the terrain of medical practice. Stemming from the biomedical model at the root of medical epistemology, this body is regarded as an object external to the enquiries which yield knowledge of it (Lyon and Barbalet, 1994: 52). This is the functioning of the body as a machine paradigm and this paradigm tends to privilege the male body. This body, whether or not it is seen to be afflicted with HIV/AIDS, is perceived as a quantifiable object. Thus it can be prodded, poked, cut open, scanned, photographed, phlebotomised, and so on, under the banner of medical science. Clearly, it has been difficult to develop a complete picture of the 'living' female, drug-using body in this disciplinary process.

Not surprisingly, when GRID (Gay Related Immune Deficiency), the precursor to HIV/AIDS, first became identified as a medical syndrome in 1981 (Patton, 1995), and before HIV/AIDS was embedded in the public's consciousness as a bona fide disease complex, GRID was linked inextricably with men, albeit a perceived 'pathological' population of men, gay men. In the mid-1980s, due to the rising cases of HIV/AIDS related to injecting drug use, the link with injecting drug users became established. Syringe or needle exchange programmes, particularly in Western Europe, were set up to provide new or clean needles and syringes to injectors (Inciardi and Harison, 2000: ix). At this juncture in the development of AIDS as a disease, as well as a social institution (Plummer, 1988: 21), women began to be increasingly infected as well as affected by the virus (Henderson, 1990: 9).

Whether or not it was unproblematic for scientific experts to extend their HIV/AIDS pathologizing to other deviant bodies, such as male and female injecting drug users and/or male and female prostitutes, may remain unclear at first glance. Needless to say in the early days of HIV/AIDS the scopic drive of biomedicine must have been in overdrive. However, the idea that male and female injecting drug users and male and female prostitutes identified as socially deviant are somatically different from 'normal' people has been a recurrent idea rooted in Western popular thought and culture (Urla and Terry, 1995: 1). Translated to biomedicine these bodies represented illness states which could arise without any physical mediation (Armstrong, 2002: 106).

From earlier discussions in this book, we know already that society's experts have a penchant for creating all sorts of deviant bodies within the regulatory regimes of medicine, science and law. Biomedical experts, in particular, construct bodies through precise investigatory techniques and culturally wedged and, at times, prejudicial research goals framed by the routines of life in a professional bureaucracy (Chambliss, 1996). Significantly, the disciplinary power of medicine with regard to HIV/AIDS has been consistently maintained through the proliferation of a public health discourse whose rhetoric implies the freedom of individuals to behave as they wish pitted against the rights of society to control individuals' bodies in the name of health (Lupton, 1994: 32). The fact that, over time, the lives of women of colour – in particular, Black women – have been victimized by substance use and HIV/AIDS (Durr, 2005: 723) is often glossed over in this rhetoric.

In this context, Jacqueline Urla and Jennifer Terry (1995: 2) suggest, in an age of killer viruses and dangerous genes, methods for finding a whole host of socially and scientifically menacing bodies are contributing to the construction of new, biologically demonized underclasses. Clearly, again we see that significant social issues are being displaced onto the body. With regard to the social issue of HIV/AIDS, the fact that white, Western, middle class, male bodies were the definitional norm with regard to HIV/AIDS meant that there was an unstable coexistence of social deviance and medical health within the body subject to this killer virus (Patton, 1995: 340). This coexistence resulted in the cultural perception that certain types of bodies, usually male, were at risk. That these bodies were identified initially as deviant men's bodies (for example, homosexuals) must not be underestimated. However misplaced, this deviant identification offered a powerful means for punishing, disciplining and controlling gay men's sexual proclivities through the biomedical gaze. This identification also allowed Gothic horror to become embedded in our public awareness through the structuring and coding of the HIV/AIDS discourse in such a way as to fend off bodies who could be identified with the virus and subsequently to view them as transgressive, abject or monstrous (Williamson, 1989: 76). Of course, these notions could be matched with particular gendered bodies. Gradually, alongside gay men's bodies, the bodies of women, particularly 'bad' women's bodies such as prostitutes, Black women, female injecting drug users and promiscuous women (Kitzinger, 1994), appeared to embody the threat of HIV/AIDS and they became transformed into transgressive, abject or monstrous bodies.

As implied above, the male-ing of HIV/AIDS has made it difficult to develop a feminist embodiment perspective. This is not only because male bodies were privileged over female bodies. It is also because when a social issue such as HIV/AIDS is displaced primarily on male bodies, other bodies affected by the disease, such as female injecting drug users, are not allowed equivalent discursive power in the fight to define the meaning of HIV/AIDS in their personal and political lives. Their embodied agency becomes obscured, as do the ways in which HIV/AIDS is constructed. While the early accounts of HIV/AIDS as a white, male gay disease have been discredited, the initial male-ing and indeed gendering of HIV/AIDS compelled us to lose sight of how notions of gender and sexuality, as well as race and class, have been and continue to be actively employed in the HIV/AIDS discourse.

In tracing the development of the HIV/AIDS discourse related to drug users, we can see the primacy of male over female bodies. For example in one study (Singer et al., 2001), male more than female drug users were found to be embroiled in 'war stories', revealing insider narratives of street experiences. On the spectrum of embodied pain, women's street narratives represented a visceral, internalized sense of suffering focused on previous experience of male violence and sexual abuse. Female bodies were consistently battered and violated, a finding confirmed in the drugs literature (Bloom, 2002; Green, et al., 2002; Evans et al., 2002; Erickson et al., 2000; Metsch et al., 1999; Wetherington and Roman, 1998; Chermack, Fuller and Blow, 2000; He et al., 1999; Mazza and Dennerstein, 1996; Stevens and Wexler, 1999; Maher, 1997; Anderson and Snow, 1998; Welle, Falkin and Jainchill, 1998; Davis and DiNitto, 1996; Sterk, 1999; Kandall, 1996).

On the other hand, men's narratives reflected experiences of social suffering and regret and were saturated with notions of fatalism and futility. Nevertheless, the ability to embody power and experience empowerment was within the reach of men's, but not women's bodies. In addition, when looking at 'strawberries' or men and women who trade sex acts for a variety of illegal drugs, researchers (Elwood et al., 1997) contend that any male, female, White, Hispanic and African American user can be at risk for 'strawberry behaviours'. However, it is clear that, in comparison to men, women are more likely to trade their bodies for drugs. The above authors suggest an interpretation based on women's access to economic resources and gender scripts in which women are considered more subordinate to men. Furthermore, although racialized bodies of Black women feature centrally in this 'story', this fact is downplayed by the authors, although they do not want their findings to discount the plight of Black 'female strawberries'. We the readers are left with the message that the conditions that lead to trading one's body for drugs transcend gender and ethnicity. Unfortunately the hidden or covert message is that trading one's body for drugs, drug use, risk-taking and HIV/AIDS transmission are interrelated in complex ways and this complexity is based on the privileging of male over female bodies. Furthermore this apparent complexity downplays the potential effects of HIV on female, in particular Black female, bodies. Where is the social justice in this message?

Here the key to developing a feminist embodiment perspective, rather than replacing female bodies with male bodies in the centre or as the norm of clinical HIV/AIDS, is the abandonment of the idea of the normative, norm or centre in this specific context, as should be the case generally in feminist politics (Bryson, 1999: 204). We don't need a new normative body based on the experiences and interests of White, middle-class women and ignoring those of other groups. What we need are theories that are anti-oppressive and which develop a sharper focus on the concepts of embodied intersectionality and multiplicity by complicating and theorizing the concept of difference (Moosa-Mitha, 2005: 63).

At this juncture, difference cannot be about favouring an essentially biological difference between the sexes (within or outside the drugs field); rather difference is concerned with the mechanisms by which bodies are recognized as different only in so far as they are constructed as possessing or lacking some socially privileged quality or qualities (Gatens, 1992: 135). We must contemplate a multiplicity of differences in the drugs field and this means that class and race are just as important as gender in terms of cultural emblems of embodied oppression.

HIV/AIDS and women's functionality vis-à-vis heterosexuality

While we have seen the centrality of male bodies in defining the HIV/AIDS discourse, let us now turn our attention to another problem that we encounter in our desire to develop a feminist embodiment approach in this area. This problem relates to women's functionality vis-à-vis heterosexuality. This sort of functionality reflects the cultural concern with constructing female sexuality around its relationship to male bodies. However, it also reflects the feminist concern with how to demand multiple ways of being in the world when woman as subject seems to have been consistently marked by heteronormativity. Let us look more closely at these issues.

Social research in the area of HIV/AIDS has been concerned with examining the ways in which risky sexual practices can be seen as part of pervasive cultural constructions of sexuality (see Weeks, 1985; Watney, 1987; Holland et al., 1998). This perspective attempts to counter the more common approach of pathologizing HIV/AIDS as a problem of specific minorities (for example, gays, drug users, young urban black people, and so on) (Brook, 1999: 66). More than twenty years ago, Simon Watney (1987: 8) contended that these three constituencies were already feared and marginalized in the West and that the presence of HIV/AIDS in these groups was perceived as not accidental but as a symbolic extension of some imagined inner embodied essence of being, manifesting itself as a disease.

While in this debate feminist research identifies women's bodies as an important part of the HIV/AIDS underclass, it becomes clear that one of the reasons for women's inclusion in this underclass has been based on male heterosexual desire, alongside the visibility of heterosexual women as a symbol of functionality or normality whether as carers or mothers (Richardson, 1996: 164). The dual impact of male heterosexual desire and the HIV/AIDS risk reduction discourse on women has meant that their bodies have been held morally and socially responsible for the control of sex and reproduction (Bell, 1992: 53). This responsibility has been translated into a form of embodied control and a way of employing technologies of the self, rendering women's bodies incapable of reproduction, whether temporarily through contraception or terminations or permanently through sterilization (Richardson, 1993). Here, in relation to men's bodies, women's bodies are perceived as more leaky (Shidrick, 1997) and open (E. Martin, 1992). Given that women's sexual organs are constructed as repositories of contamination, heterosexual women in particular are represented as more potentially infecting or polluting than heterosexual men and the burden of responsibility is placed on their bodies for protecting both themselves and their partners from HIV infection (Lupton, 1999: 141). Acutely aware of this imbalance, researchers (Stevens, Tortu and Coyle, 1998: 22) have noted that more attention needs to be paid to the role of the male drug injector in heterosexual transmission of HIV to combat the tendency to place responsibility on women.

But this type of responsibility on women for providing protection or risk reduction with regard to heterosexual men has come through cultural, scientific and normative directives that focus on female bodies as their targets and as being more dangerous or precarious than men's bodies. In this context, Braidotti (1994: 42) notes that with the contraceptive pill we have sex without babies and with the new reproductive technologies we have babies without sex. For her, an added factor is that as contraception and the new reproductive technologies have arisen vis-à-vis women's bodies, the AIDS epidemic has been manipulated by patriarchal conservatism and marketed so as to carry a clear and simple message that 'Sex kills'. Of course in this complex social and cultural process, normative male heterosexuality is privileged as women's bodies are further disciplined and controlled. If sex kills, women kill because their bodies have become the metaphor for sexuality (Davis, 1997: 5).

Within this sort of patriarchal conservatism, women's bodies have been shaped as affective, emotional bodies 'in relation to the other/others' rather than as embodying autonomy or moral agency. These female bodies are rooted in base corporeality 'in themselves' rather than 'for themselves', which means their exclusion from full rationality, a parameter of moral agency (Shildrick, 1997: 81). Thus not having real control over their bodies women are seen to play a functional, affective role vis-à-vis the sexual economy of 'rational' heterosexuality. The fact that women's bodies have been perceived as being weak, fragile and easily damaged has historically served to support policies excluding women from a variety of social goods (Sheldon, 2002: 14). With regard to HIV/AIDS, this can be translated into barring women from needed treatment and health care. Significantly, the only noteworthy interest in women in the research effort on HIV/AIDS concerned women's potential as 'vectors' to infect others, either as sexual partners, especially as polluted, prostituting bodies or as vessels or gestators – reproductive bodies (Faden, Kass and McGraw, 1996: 252–3) with maternal possibilities. Alternatively, women were ignored altogether by the research community.

It is not surprising that these sorts of ideas embedded in popular culture have been translated into the world of illegal drugs where we find that kinship, relationality and orientation towards others appear to be inscribed on women drug user's risky bodies. For example, researchers (Riess, Kim and Downing, 2001) found, when looking at motives for HIV testing in frequently mentioned categories, that female more than male injecting drug users considered others in their decision-making framework. Women more than men took into account the financial benefits for themselves, as well as their families, were motivated to find out their HIV status with regard to concerns related to family and significant others and wanted to be able to make an informed decision about the possibility of transmitting HIV to a newborn.

In a related context, other researchers (Sherman, Latkin and Gielen, 2001) look at women's sometimes risky needle-sharing behaviour within the context of HIV/AIDS. Here I would like to take a slight diversion. I have always been fascinated by the notion of 'sharing' needles and syringes in the drug-using community. In my mind it is an odd notion, given that society implicates drug users in engaging in an immoral activity while at the same time attributing to them the moral capability of sharing with others. How is this possible? Perhaps this reflects a clear way in which HIV/AIDS as a disease is changing the drugs field and demonstrates that deviant bodies can also be moral bodies. But of course morality in the drugs world is gendered as well as defined by how well women share not only their needles but their bodies with men. For women, any form of sexual difference, such as lesbianism, bisexuality, intersexuality and being transgendered (Lombardi and Van Servellen, 2000; Ettorre, 2005b), which is counter to heteronormativity is shunned.

If we return to the topic of women's sometimes risky needle sharing, we see through the work of the above mentioned authors (Sherman, Latkin and Gielen, 2001) that women injecting drug users may be sharing their needles and syringes more often than men and with a larger proportion of their social network members. This finding was explained as a consequence of women's overall social and support networks being significantly larger than men's, as well as the nature of women's relationships within the drug-using world: women had a larger percentage of sex partners and kin. Here, women's more than men's bodies become inscribed by risk because of kin and 'otherness' in the wide expanse of their social environment. If technologies of the self, such as using clean needles, employing safe sex through condoms and injecting drugs, are employed, women's bodies are thought to be treading on safer ground.

Women drug users will thus be seen to be more self-disciplined. However, sexuality and reproduction as the targets of biopower ultimately discipline women's bodies. With regard to their drug use, biopower's range becomes far reaching as it affects their risky, gendered bodies' deployment as well as the non-deployment of these technologies of self. For women who abuse drugs, embodying self-discipline may have a relational, health and cultural value. But they are often vulnerable to a type of heteronormativity which demands giving over their seemingly receptive bodies to men, regardless of whether or not this reflects their real desires or needs. Thus it is not surprising to find that women who use drugs participate in risky sexual practices and are more likely than men to develop an HIV infection from receptive sex as well as sharing of needles (Tardiff et al., 1997). We should be aware in this context that drug use, sexuality and risk are subject to regulation and control through a multiplicity of institutions, each with their own discursive practices and textual strategies (McRobbie, 1995: 185). The drug world, gender, HIV/AIDS, medicine, reproduction, the law, and so on, are all regulatory regimes in which we can find disciplinary practices and cultural mechanisms by which different bodies are constructed as advantaged or not. Set alongside the heterosexual matrix (Butler, 1990), women's sexual materiality, particularly in the drugs field, may or may not place them at a disadvantage. But the sense of relationality and links with 'kith and kin' which are imputed to their bodies in the drugs field may be hard for them to shake off physically, sexually and culturally.

Contesting the link between prostitution and drug use or why the 'whore, drugs and risk cultural configuration' doesn't work

When looking at the HIV/AIDS discourse through the lens of female embodiment, we find an assumption, particularly in the drugs field, that female drug users will usually engage in prostitution to support their illegal drugs habit. The link between prostitution and illegal drug use for women was upheld consistently for many years prior to the emergence of HIV/AIDS. This link is established regardless of the fact that the empirical evidence to support these claims, in my view, tends to be lacking. Thus claims such as these remain over-determined. Consistently the implication in the drugs field is that if a woman is a prostitute she will use drugs and be at risk of HIV or if she is a drug user she will be a prostitute, and so on. This 'whore, drugs and risk' cultural configuration sets up cultural representations of women who put their bodies on a sex market, as those women whose lives embody drug use as a permanent fixture. These cultural beliefs are set up against an economy of drug use which defines these prostitutes by their transgressive, deviant possibilities in an epidemiologic framework in which the individualization of risk is predominant (Buchanan et al., 2003). On the other hand, these beliefs confront a politics of the body in these hazardous cultures where risk is constructed as a socially and culturally organized phenomenon rather than an individual one (Rhodes, 1997; Rhodes and Stimson, 1994).

Here there needs to be a shift of intellectual terrain from thinking about prostitution and its link with drugs and unsafe sex to women's bodies in sex-exchange situations themselves and all sorts of embodied risks, hazardous practices, or frightening prospects, such as murder, violence, homelessness, police harassment, exploitation, ill health, loss of children, poverty, crime, and so on – all of which arise in these risky situations. Much work in the drugs field presents prostitution and drugs as an inevitable material fact of our cultural life (see, for example, Vaarwerk and Gaal, 2001; McKeganey, 2006; McKeganey and Barnard, 1996; McKeganey et al., 1992). These researchers appear to accept unquestioningly that a prostitute, sex worker or woman who exchanges her body or bodily performances for money will be using drugs and thus will be at risk of HIV/AIDS. Also, these researchers assume that a prostitute's ability to be visible on a sex-exchange market is the foundation of prostitution and that a drugs market will inevitably be close by, if not intertwined with this sex market.

Such a view takes prostitutes' drug using as a self-explanatory primary cause and awards it an impenetrable and horrifying facticity. In turn, this inhibits our ability and, in some cases, our desire to contest or discredit this view of prostitution's link with drugs use. To view drug use and prostitution as inexorably linked obscures the fact that expensive drug use and poverty may propel women into illegal work careers, such as shoplifting, sex work and drug dealing (Murphy and Rosenbaum, 1999: 46), and that their social connections are not constrained by geographical boundaries: simply, drug users are a mobile population (McCoy, Correa and Fritz, 1996).

Indeed, becoming a prostituting drug user or a drug-using prostitute can be a response to limited conventional opportunities (May et al., 1999: 5) and social circumstances typified by a narrowing of life's options that decreases one's ability to assume conventional roles (Mullings, Marquart and Diamond, 2001). Furthermore, while sex may be commodified for these women, the dominant view of commodified sex as wholly oppositional to intimate romantic relations is not only mistaken but also somewhat of a cultural contradiction; these commodified sexual relations are not homogeneous; they can be romantic and forms of sexual exchange and these exchanges are not particular to low income and drug-using women (Mulia, 2000: 742). Furthermore these exchanges can appear to embody risk and trust (Davis et al., 1997). However, acknowledging risks and anxieties about HIV/AIDS in these everyday contexts is difficult exactly because it calls trust and intimacy into question (Holland et al., 1992: 277).

To treat drug-using women as prostituting women or prostituting women as drug-using women can mean that to consider prostitution and drug use as separate issues is beyond our grasp. In its efforts to explore the difficulties with women's drug-using and prostituting bodies and perhaps to express a certain level of pity, if not sympathy, for these women, this sort of approach coincides with a masculinist culture which organizes, frames and relegates these female bodies to a discourse of risk where HIV/AIDS is constructed as a behavioural disease (Stimson, 1990). The implication is that whether one is a prostituting body or a drug-using body, a female body is pressed into the service of harm reduction, as well as constructed as a risky body, subject to punishment for bad behaviour and potential leakiness. She is seen as one who will automatically transmit HIV/AIDS. In other words, she will not practice safer sex with her male customers or punters. It is difficult here to have a true picture of the risk practices of prostitutes (Cusick, Martin and May, 2003). Although substance use increases sexual risk taking, women who use substances are more likely to use safe sex practices than women who don't (Sly and Riehman, 1999). However, drug-using women report higher levels of risk than men (Stevens, Estrada and Estrada, 1998) and crack cocaine–using women reported having unprotected sex in exchange for drugs (Cross et al., 2001).

Regardless of the above, when will we break the intractable link that is continuously made by researchers between female prostituting bodies and female drug-using bodies? A rupturing of this link is required and in turn this rupturing demands a certain amount of flexibility in our approach to female drug-using bodies. Most certainly it demands, as implied earlier, a move toward theorizing difference and interrogating the normative assumptions and practices that exist both in marginalized and privileged spaces in the drug-using world and drug-research field. Obviously the spaces filled by female prostitutes, as well as female drug users, are marginalized, disciplinary spaces seen to be populated by all sorts of deviant diseased bodies. We need to give space both theoretically and empirically to these bodies so that we can see them more clearly than we do now.

Here I would contend that this type of considered feminist approach is urgently needed in the drugs field as, more often than not, masculinist spaces are viewed not only as privileged spaces reflecting masculine hegemony (Collison, 1996), but also as the reflexive situatedness from where most if not all theorizing in the drugs field emanates. We know that within the realm of the embodied practice of injecting drugs women's need for harm reduction may not be fully addressed (Miller et al., 2001). Nevertheless we must ensure that women no longer emerge as second-class drug users, as well as having more contaminated, polluted bodies than men.

Women drug users' bodies and the postmodern moment of HIV/AIDS

In this chapter, I have attempted to clarify the problems which hinder the development of a feminist-embodiment approach to drugs and HIV/AIDS. We looked closely at three, somewhat intractable problems which have clogged up our theorizing. With these problems in mind, I demonstrated how we need to build up a flexible approach in the area, meaning that we need to theorize difference on multiple levels.

At this historical juncture, HIV/AIDS has enabled instances in our culture for us to have a close look at death. The spread of HIV/AIDS is a recent and powerful reminder of the threat of the body (Hallam, Hockey and Howarth, 1999: 125) and its dangerous potential. Of course, we knew the dangers of the drug-using body well before HIV/AIDS came on the scene, as well as recognized it as a site of pollution, disease and disorder, as well as pleasure and consumption. Yet we now have an added awareness shaped by the horror and dread that our culture has betrayed us.

In this context, John O'Neill (2001: 181) contends that nothing represents the postmodern moment in our history more vividly than the transformation of our sexuality in its encounter with the HIV/AIDS virus. The combination of the fear that our lovemaking threatens to kill us and the knowledge that biomedicine has not come up with a cure for HIV/AIDS means that we are abandoned to *horror autotoxicus* (that is, the catastrophe of bodily fluids being lethal and dealing death). O'Neill (2001: 181) goes on further to say that we should not speak of persons with AIDS but rather of a society with AIDS, a society in which AIDS connotes the complex of psychosocial, legal, economic and political responses to persons with HIV and its related diseases. What John O'Neill (2001: 181) pinpoints is the often hidden reality that AIDS is all about how society responds to itself. This response is affected by the recently acquired knowledge that the auto-immunity which functioned as an assurance of principles of sexual freedom, and which 'society' believed it took pleasure in as an advanced medicalized one, is an illusion. Furthermore, in contemporary society's response to itself the notion of itself as a well-functioning political community is lost, given that the peril of HIV/AIDS carves us up according to the politics of pollution, disease, crime and desire.

In conclusion, we can ask: What sense of optimism are women drug users able to have in this postmodern moment? How does the *'horror autotoxicus'* affect their bodies? Briefly I want to reflect on some of Rosi Braidotti's (2002) ideas in looking for answers to these questions. Rather than focusing on melancholia and mourning in this postmodern moment, Braidotti (2002: 53) emphasizes pleasure as a constitutive element of subjectivity. I think the challenge we in the drugs field face today is to focus more on pleasure and human fulfilment in our quest for bodily integrity in the face of the threats it faces. In the midst of these troubling times, we need hopeful metaphors – we need to hold on to what matters. For example, Betania Allen (2006), in her study of Mexican women with HIV/AIDS, showed how these women developed encouraging subaltern theories of health which not only challenged positively hegemonic biomedical thinking but also allowed them to transform their illness experiences to more hopeful ones which embodied psychological health. Patti Lather (1999) in her work on women affected with HIV/AIDS demonstrates how lack of health became for many of these women an enabling condition. The notion of positive women was double-edged, reflecting a body inscribed by HIV/AIDS, as well as one processing information as an optimistic woman (see also Lather and Smithies, 1997).

In our drug-using society with HIV/AIDS, we need more female and indeed male bodies who embrace this double-edged positivity. Furthermore we need to ensure that the mechanisms and practices by which gendered, raced and classed bodies are recognized as different and contaminated by HIV/AIDS begin to possess social privilege and are allowed to experience a sense of social justice.

8
Embodiment, Emotions and Female Drug Use

> The study of female mass movements calls attention to female consciousness. It is possible to examine a range of motivations in the everyday lives of women that might lead them collectively in pursuit of goals they could not attain as individuals. Women's movements follow common patterns: they focus on consumer and peace issues and they oppose outside aggressors. Accepting and enforcing the division of labour by sex, therefore, can bring women into conflict with authorities. Women may even attack their rulers when food prices rise too high for suspicious reasons, when sexual harassment brings women's dignity into question, or when the community of women appears to be under attack... A sense of community that emerges from shared routines binds women to one another within their class and within their neighborhoods... Physical proximity – such as occurs in plazas, wash houses, markets, church entries, beauty parlors and even female jails – contributes to the power of female community. These loose networks facilitate the tight bonds that exhibit their strength in times of collective action.
>
> Temma Kaplan (1982: 57)

Fitting in the emotionality piece

Thus far in this book we have built up a feminist embodiment approach to drugs and looked at some of the different types of embodiment that are on offer to drug-using women. Wanting to revision, we let go of how we have traditionally seen women and drug use and attempted to construct new perceptions of women's drug-using bodies. I have maintained this type of focus to challenge some of the hurtful, biased and obsolete images of and approaches to women drug users that are in circulation at the moment, and to construct new understandings which are positive and empowering rather than moralistic and destructive. In doing so, I have attempted to construct images and representations that are grounded in the bodies of real drug-using women, no matter how these female bodies differ from one another in terms of race, ethnicity, class, age, ability, and so on.

However, one more piece of the women and drugs use issue needs to be inserted into the embodiment puzzle, and that 'piece' is emotionality, embodied emotions or what we see as emerging from the affective dimensions of gendered drug use – an issue which I touched upon in Chapter 3 when I discussed briefly women drug users' 'cultures of emotions'. In this chapter, I want to extend that previous discussion and examine emotions side by side women's drug-using bodies. Here my basic assumption is that the study of emotions requires a conception of the human body as a lived structure of ongoing experience and that emotions entail both embodied feelings and cognitive orientations, public morality and cultural ideology, while providing a missing link capable of bridging mind and body, individual, society and body politic (Williams and Bendelow, 1998: 137).

Focusing on emotions in this way, we begin to fashion a needed 'non-dualistic ontology of the mindful body in which emotions play a central role in the human experience and cultural scripts of health, sickness, disability and death' (Williams and Bendelow, 1996: 47) and, I would add, risk. In considering emotions as central to human embodiment, I would like to consider further how emotions have a central part to play in the morality of gendered, drug-using bodies, regardless of how these bodies are shaped and appear within public discourses.

Before those of us concerned with the issue of women, the body and drug use are able to grasp the complexity of these embodiment issues, we should have an understanding of the answers to the following, essential questions: (i) How does the emotional economy of women relate to women drug users and how does this economy become embodied? (ii) In what areas do those who study emotion agree and how does it connect to the emotional embodiment of women drug users? (iii) How are we able to demonstrate that the affective dimensions of risk are culturally dependent 'embodied processes'? (iv) Within this discussion, what types of feminist strategies are needed both collectively and individually for women drug users to achieve successful embodiment? These questions will be answered in the following discussions.

How does the emotional economy of women relate to women drug users and how does this economy become embodied?

Earlier, we saw that as a form of 'embodied deviance', drug use 'marks' bodies of individuals and determines their low social status and lack of moral agency. We also saw that a drug-using body becomes a vehicle for solving a variety of problems that all bodies must face. But these problems, including restraint, representation, regulation and reproduction, become magnified and more complicated when race, gender and class are powerfully inscribed on bodies, making them different one from another (see Chapter 2 for a full discussion of these bodily tasks). I have chosen specifically to focus on gender and, more specifically, the gendering of female bodies because I see some cultural and social differences between the problem of female and male drug use, as I have argued in my previous work (Ettorre, 1989a and b, 1992, 1994, 2004).

In my view, the problem of female drug use and the symptoms that are constructed around this problem disclose themselves as a 'textuality'. For example, severe mental illness (DiNitto, Webb and Rubin, 2002); mental health problems and perceived obstacles to working, such as stigma, fear of failure and insufficient skills (Laudet et al., 2002); women drug users' more benign form of schizophrenia in comparison to men (Gearon and Bellack, 2000); and stress, chronic illnesses and psychological disorders that develop from an unhealthy lifestyle (Miley, 2001) are just a few of the problems which have symbolic significance in the drugs field. All of these socially constructed problems are representative of the cultural and social differences between the problems of female and male drug use.

These and other similar symptoms and troubles linked to female drug use have political significance under the shifting rules governing the historical construction of gender. Inevitably, the body of any female sufferer is deeply inscribed with an ideological construction of femininity emblematic at any particular historical moment. This implies that the bodies of disordered women, such as drug users, offer themselves up to the social interpreter to be read as a cultural statement about gender and the rules for the cultural constructions of femininity (Bordo, 1993a:168). According to these rules, women need to develop a totally other-oriented emotional economy (Bordo, 1993a: 171).

In this other-oriented emotional economy, regulation of the female use of psychotropic or mind-altering substances operates and this type of use is frowned upon. This regulation and cultural control of women reveals the wide-ranging rule governing the construction of femininity – that the female need to be wild, fierce, rowdy and uncontrollable, to have pleasure and fun or to express female desire (Hinchcliff, 2000), even in the midst of the difficulties of poverty and ethnic discrimination (Valdez, Kaplan and Cepeda, 2000) must be restricted or limited. Moreover in this other-oriented emotional economy the control of women's behaviour is paramount, as is her own self-discipline. A woman must always be seen to be in control of her desires and to reject illegal drugs or else she risks contaminating morals, babies and families, as well as her body. Consistently, female desire must be regulated and self-supervised, as well as oriented towards the other/s, not oneself.

What this means on an embodiment level for any woman is that her female body, the deployment of her emotions and the enactment of her desires must be primarily for others and not for herself. A woman's most important emotional experiences must be seen to be based on others. Women's bodies become conduits of others' emotional lives, whether this is expressed through kinship, normative heterosexual desire or procreation. Their bodies can be represented as cultural vessels through which, in which and by which intimacy passes through and, as a result, these vessels are revered (Faden, Kass and McGraw, 1996). Of course, this applies primarily to non-drug-using women.

The problem for female drug users is that the notion of cultural containers of intimacy not only bypasses them but also is inaccessible to them. Their bodies represent defilement and contamination, not reverence. They are not worthy of intimacy or close relationships. However, if they have intimate 'normative' relations these may be troublesome, albeit sexually reciprocal (Mulia, 2000) and most definitely influenced by culture and class.

In this context, some researchers (Newcomb and Rickards, 1995) have argued that being raised by drug-abusing parents may create for their children problems with intimacy in later life and family support is strongly associated with good adult intimate relations. Of course, what this really means is that parental drug users, especially female ones, are perceived as being unable to provide appropriate family support and will be blamed for causing their children's intimacy problems. While the issue of restriction of desire is central to the emotional economy of female drug users and explains a lot about why they appear to be more stigmatized and punished in comparison to their male counterparts, their embodiment is represented as those contaminated or polluted vessels/bodies which appear to have lost their basic human right to intimacy.

In what areas do those who study emotion agree and how does it link to the emotional embodiment of women drug users?

Despite the idea in popular culture that drug users have an almost in-built compulsion to take drugs, there needs to be some form of emotional engagement on a bodily level which moves them. For the following discussion, I am reliant on the illuminating work of feminist thinkers Renee Anspach and Diane Beeson (2001: 113–16) who outline four key areas where students of emotions agree and whose work places emotions centrally in the sphere of medical and moral life. For these feminist authors, students of emotions agree on the following four precepts: emotions are a way of knowing; emotions are socially and culturally constructed; emotions are ineluctably tied to power relations; and emotions are fundamental ingredients of moral life. While these authors recognize the importance of embodiment vis-à-vis emotions, their main concern is to consider the ethical implications of emotions within a feminist approach and to delineate how emotional experiences are shaped by cultural, social and institutional arrangements. In this context, I am keen to look at each precept in turn and to make connections with drug users, specifically female drug users and their emotional embodiment. Consequently, I will suggest a need for embodied ethics in the drugs field.

Emotions as a way of knowing

Here Anspach and Beeson (2001: 113–4) contend that emotions themselves can be a legitimate foundation of knowledge. In this context, they suggest that emotions are instrumental in helping us to judge social reality, find out about our cultural and social worlds and analyse the workings of the social bond in which we are complicit. Emotions can be public displays as well as relational displays and there can be endless ways of making these displays of emotions visible in popular culture. For example, think of Lady Diana's death and the public displays of grief in Britain, as well as relational displays of love enacted in heterosexual marriages or lesbian and gay civil partnerships.

The key point here is that emotion, as the feeling of bodily change (Ahmed, 2004: 5) allows us to get in touch with the world around us as well as our changeable, sentient bodies which respond to that world. Through our emotions we become knowledgeable about how society and bodies work, have access to the complex web of social relationships that is society, are able to retrieve the sometimes submerged feelings which emerge in our interactions with others and direct our bodies in ways which reflect feelings of corporeal changes. Additionally, particularly for those who are excluded on the basis of 'difference' from the norm of white, Western, masculinist society, emotion can act as an important gauge, measuring social injustice.

For drug users, emotions are obviously very significant because it is through the feeling of bodily change, whether it is experienced as pleasurable or painful, that the pursuit of drugs becomes one's embodied habit. The practices and technologies of drug use are deeply embodied and it is through the repetition of these practices and technologies of use that the drug-using body materializes. A drug is taken, the feeling of bodily change occurs and one gains access into the somewhat invisible world of drug use and the bodily cycle goes on. For female drugs users, feeling ashamed and contaminated or dirty become 'mates' to culture's indignation and fear. We know that affect regulation is significant in the healing process for female drug users and an awareness of this type of affect regulation can enable them to deal with feelings of being dirty, afraid or worthless (Millar & Stermac, 2000). Thus, for female drug users cultivating positive emotions and focusing on affect allows them to have access to a new sense of embodiment other than drug taking and to know more about the affective dimensions of a non-drug-using life style.

Emotions as socially and culturally constructed

In this context, Anspach and Beeson (2001) note that the emphasis on the relationship of emotions to cultural and social arrangements may vary for social theorists, but there is a general consensus that emotions reproduce customary forms of social and cultural life and these emotions are historically dependent and culturally changeable. Indeed, Ahmed (2004: 34) speaks about the histories of emotions and how, for instance, pain is not merely an effect of a history of harm but also the 'bodily life of that history'. When we consider bodily lives within the context of histories of emotions, we must also keep clearly within our frame the cultural constructions of gendered bodies side by side their own emotional histories.

In particular, the female body is the gendered body which is seen to be ruled by emotions. This body becomes a metaphor for the body pole of the mind/body dualism, 'representing nature, irrationality and sensuality', in contrast to the mind or 'masculine will', the normalized position of 'social power, rationality and self-control' (Davis, 1997: 5). In this binary narrative, experts in the drug field perpetuate gender stereotypes. In effect, women's drug-using bodies may represent emotions in the moral economy of drug use. However, their negative emotions will become exacerbated on the street scene when their bodily scars and physical damage from drug using make them 'feel like garbage', exposing the symbolic violence contained in the moral anatomy of their own drug-using bodies (Epele, 2002). The effects are that while women's bodies may be seen as carrying more emotions than men's in the drugs world, these female bodies are targets of hate and derision more often than men's. Furthermore, evidence of drug use is literally inscribed upon their bodies through scarring, and so on, having the potential to make these women full of self-hate, if not shame. These female drug users have failed in their bodily task of representation, and in the end their bodies become a source of embarrassment, if not disgrace to them.

Emotions as ineluctably tied to power relations

Ascriptions of emotions can serve as potent tools for domination and social control (Anspach and Beeson; 2001: 114). One way to disempower, discredit or discount those who are 'different' in society is to label them as 'irrational' which can translate to mean 'emotional'. As the above authors suggest, emotionality is most likely to be attributed to dominated groups in society. Against the backdrop of emotions, the narratives of dominated groups may detail certain physiological changes that occur, the embodied choices that they make and the participatory framework in which these are set. But when one feels with one's body, there is always emotional work to be done. In this respect, one's personal and public emotions, as well as shared experiences of bodily feelings, will inevitably be disciplined and controlled by larger political processes which will, at times, dwarf this emotional work. The entirety of the political disciplining that goes into this process is incalculable.

For drug users, their emotions are very often shaped in response to the practical and technical knowledge, judgements and authority of the experts. 'Becoming clean' is perceived as a time of intense emotional labour when one's body is pressed into the service of the drug treatment industry. The problem for female drug users is that while they may 'become clean', their emotional competence is often judged in relationship to their social competence which is found to be lacking or significantly lower than male drug users (Rutherford et al., 1997). In effect, for some female drug users, healing may be experienced as a failure in social skills and emotional fitness, an experience which can have devastating repercussions in their lives, especially for those in traditional forms of treatment who are pregnant or have children (Nishimoto and Roberts, 2001).

Emotions as fundamental ingredients of moral life

Rather than seeing emotions as an obstacle to rationality, emotions and cultural values are inexorably linked (Anspach and Beeson, 2001: 115). These authors argue further that we take satisfaction in social practices that we appraise positively and are humiliated by those we appraise negatively. The sociality of emotions – the conditional link of being with others – requires an ethics that begins with your emotions and moving towards you and getting close enough to touch you and perhaps for you to feel the trace of the emotion on your body (Ahmed, 2004: 31).

Here I argue that while our emotions are embodied, so also are our ethics (see Ettorre, 2002: 123–34) and these are linked as moral inscriptions are made on the body. As suggested by Sara Ahmed (2004), emotions are inscribed on our bodies by the very fact that we are in relation to others. We are able to experience the feeling of bodily change for others within ourselves and this represents moral behaviour. In this context, our embodied ethics should be based on emotions and the principle of responsibility. This means that, as human subjects, we are grounded in inter-subjectivity and through inter-subjectivity or our relationships with others, we 'are capable of hearing and responding to the call of the other' (Martin 1992: 305). As Zygmunt Bauman (1993: 90) suggests: 'I am responsible for the Other's condition; but being responsible in a responsible way, being responsible for my responsibility demands that I know what that condition is'.

How can we hear the voice of the other, if the other is dominated or voiceless? By what means will the other be heard? In asking these sorts of questions, I see drug users in this type of voiceless position, given that society disempowers drug users and does not take satisfaction in their drug use. On the contrary, drug use is judged negatively and drug users are humiliated by those negative appraisals as well as our lack of knowing what their 'condition' really is. Given the exclusionary practices directed towards drug users, the general sociality of emotions, which is purported to be experienced by 'normal' (that is, non-drug-using) people, becomes blocked when these emotions concern drug users. The common cultural urge is to move away rather than towards drug users – to shun them and exclude them from normative culture. It could be argued that this type of moralising has the effect of intensifying their emotional levels of feeling sad, guilty and ashamed, while female drug users who tend to be judged as more immoral than male drug users (Ettorre, 1992) are left feeling more depressed or sad (Meehan et al., 1996), as well as desperate.

How are we able to demonstrate that the affective dimensions of risk are culturally dependent 'embodied processes' for drug users?

In analysing what can be seen as risk identities, such as those of drug users, we need to contextualize embodiment in cultural and political terms and as politically inscribed. We need to keep in mind that bodies' biologies, physiologies and cultural narratives are shaped within historical moments and practices of suppression and restraint, as well as difference, risk and emotions.

In looking at the affective dimensions of drug use, let us revisit briefly the four body questions that we asked in Chapter 2 and make links with our current discussion on emotions. For example, with regard to the question, How do I learn to control my bodily functions such as sexual desire, excretion, eating?, we saw that drug-using bodies are marked or stigmatized and these bodies are forced outside the 'limits' of 'normal' society. We also saw that compliance within the context of complex gendering processes marks both female and male bodies in risky drug-using cultures. But restraint requires rules about the kinds of feelings appropriate to particular situations. When drug users are viewed as out of control, as is often the case, they not only appear to have broken these rules but also appear to want to make a conscious split between their bodies and emotions by losing control through drugs. For female drug users, feeling self-possessed may be inaccessible to them or far from their corporeal grasp, given culture's disciplinary response of repugnance directed towards their polluted bodies.

When asking the question, How do I present myself in an acceptable way to society?, we saw that drug users' narratives were shaped by an embodied sense of personal and social agency and that these social expressions of personal agency were gendered. Agency was very present for male bodes, shaped by heroic or hedonistic identities, while it was largely lacking for females who experienced their drug use as being at the mercy of personalized, inner drives. It is hard to present oneself as 'normal' when one is consistently told or has the feeling one is not. This is how drug users experience their embodiment. In particular, female drug users have the option of presenting themselves as normal, but challenging deviant embodiment may have the effect of feeling frustrated, if not worthless in the eyes of society.

With regard to the question, How do bodies regulate themselves when they confront a variety of social problems related to urban life?, we saw drug taking being perceived as a threat to the integrity of urban life, while being a fundamental part of urban consumption. We know that both female and male users have active roles when regulating their drug behaviour in risky bodily routines. However, when these active drug-using bodies confront discipline and order in society, they may find that their drug-using motives are questioned as those in authority designate their drug-using bodies as embodying deviance and having something wrong with them – an addiction. Emotional turmoil may ensue, as happens when a human being is the target of social moralizing. Of course, given the double standard in the drugs field, the effects of this process on female drug users may be feelings of losing one's self-worth.

When asking the question, How do drug-using bodies reproduce?, we became aware that for drug users making a decision to reproduce is overlaid with ideologies concerning what sorts of bodies should reproduce. Drug-using bodies do not fall within those seen as highly reproductive for a variety of moral and medical reasons. In my mind, I envisage drug-using bodies' response to this disciplining process as one of deep sadness, especially for women. Who has the cultural right to determine which bodies should reproduce and which bodies should not? Embodied pain, sadness and disappointment emerge in this context.

Given the above discussion on emotions and the four bodily tasks vis-à-vis our analysis of risky, gendered drug-using bodies, I would like to reiterate a refrain made throughout this text, that we need to place the body at the centre of our theorizing. Drug-using bodies need to be seen as sites where narratives of risk, identity, knowledge and enactments of emotions and bodily management converge. One difficulty is that this work needs to be done with the explicit intention of demonstrating how the affective dimensions of risk are culturally dependent embodied and gendered processes. As emphasized in earlier contexts in this book, there is a need for a resurrection of the body in our work and the breathing of 'epistemological' life back into our neglected frames. Our work is about the affirmation of corporeality – making the distinct assertion that the body and specifically embodied emotions exist as a vital consideration in the drug-use discourse. In looking further at embodied risks in the gendering of drug identities, we see the body as the place where we organize tasks of self-control, self-image, regulation and reproduction. Bodies are *not* a gender-neutral system; they are shaped by gender and embodied emotions. In making these assertions, I want to reinforce the complexities of drug use, risk taking, emotions and gender.

Within this discussion, what types of feminist strategies are needed both collectively and individually for women drug users to achieve successful embodiment?

Thus far in this book we have developed a sense that embodiment issues are feminist issues because these sorts of issues help us to reconsider, rename and 're-form' the female subject. As Rosi Braidotti (1994: 158) elaborates so eloquently, we need to 'recode the female subject not as yet another sovereign, hierarchical and exclusionary subject but rather as a multiple, open ended, interconnected entity . . . we need to emphasize a vision of thinking, knowing subject as not one but rather as being split over and over again in a rainbow of yet uncoded and ever so beautiful possibilities'.

Framed by these ideas on female embodiment, our discussions in this chapter have flagged up the beautiful and sometimes not so beautiful possibilities that are available to women drug users' embodied emotions or feelings of bodily change. With this in mind, I'd like to focus very briefly on the types of embodiment strategies that are available to women drug users as they confront all sorts of embodied emotions.

What will be offered below represents a tentative and exploratory discussion of the development of embodiment strategies in our field of study. Given what we have previously discussed, we hopefully share a reflective sense that a feminist approach to women, drug use and the body is well worth exploring and developing, and furthermore this process has political implications. Let us determine the underpinning of this type of politics and envisage how a feminist approach has the potential to effect a creative response for women drug users whose bodies are viewed in varying degrees as polluted, disordered, contaminated, not worthy of bearing children, and so on.

With this as our starting point, I want to continue our study of emotions which acknowledges that emotion, as the feeling of bodily change, entails a mixture of gendering processes, embodied sensations, cognitive orientations, public ethics and cultural ideology. My contention is that specific embodiment strategies are needed for an increased awareness of female embodiment, drug use and emotions. I want to consider a series of four key strategies, including: challenging dependency while embracing it; risking reproduction; privileging pollution; and embodying pleasure. By briefly considering these four strategies, the discussion explores further the social and cultural implications of the intersections between embodied emotions and drugs and considers this issue within the context of feminist ways of thinking.

Challenging dependency while embracing it

In Chapter 3, I noted that women's dependency must be understood in cultural, economic, social and political contexts as multi-pervasive. I detailed the tandem definitions of 'dependency' and discussed the subtle and complicated implications of these dual meanings for women drug users. Now I want to politicize dependency and suggest that by challenging dependency while at the same time embracing it, female drug users can allow themselves some scope for change. For example, it is important for a woman drug user to keep in the forefront of her mind that all women, including herself, are socialized into dependency and still to consider what this means on a bodily level. A question arises in this context, 'How can her drug-using body which is perceived as an addictive body, as well as a body which has failed to be dependable to others, become a dependable body?'

The answer may vary among women drug users, but in my mind this question relates to overcoming embodied shame, which is related to feeling bad about 'failing loved others' (Ahmed, 2004: 107) and I would add 'oneself'. In this context of shame, Sara Ahmed (2004: 107) points out that showing my shame in my failure to live up to a social ideal means that I come closer to that which I have been exposed as failing. She also suggests that shame can be restorative when the shamed other can show that her failure to measure up to a social ideal is both witnessed by others and temporary. For a woman drug user, the failure of not having a good enough female or dependable body may generate shame. Through experiencing shame, she comes close to her non-dependable body. At the same time, she is embracing dependency by recognizing her shame which is witnessed by others whom she is dependent upon. As a shamed other, she can be allowed and allow herself to re-enter the family or community, as long as she recognizes that shame is temporary. Here, as we saw earlier, dependency shifts in meaning for Black ethnic minority and indigenous women drug users and their experience of shame mixes with terror as their point of entry to dependency. However, both shame and terror must also be temporary for these women if dependency is to be challenged as well as embraced.

Risking reproduction

In earlier work, I discussed feminist strategies for women in the more general context of women and substance use (Ettorre, 1992: 137–44). In that prior context, I noted seizing the means of reproduction as a key strategy. Of course, times have moved on and I am focusing more on embodiment in the current context. Nevertheless, there still needs to be an awareness of the division between the public and private for women drug users to develop a thoughtful approach to reproduction. The notion of the reproductive body has featured throughout this text. Also, as we have seen, specifically when we discussed the bodily task of reproduction (see Chapter 2), drug users, particularly female ones, are not perceived as highly reproductive for a variety of socially constructed, moral and medical reasons.

Drug use has consistently been viewed as damaging to the regulatory regime of reproduction, as well as women's reproducing bodies. Women drug users must embrace the risk of reproduction if they are to challenge the popular belief that their drug use damages the institution of reproduction and their babies. While this statement is not meant to deny the harm that drugs can cause to fetuses during pregnancy, it is meant to emphasize that much of this 'damage' is really about cultural damage to women drug users themselves. In other words, the cultural belief that women drug users are lethal fetal containers needs to be challenged.

Here embodied anger or rage is the appropriate and just emotional response for women drug users who may or may not sense that they, like all women, have a basic human right to reproduce. Of course, the discourse of emotions used in prenatal contexts with female drug users has been used politically to disempower and discredit these women. Women drug users need to learn how to read their own embodied pain as attempts are made to disempower them and to take their right to reproduce away. Part of this reading may well be expressed in an embodied rage that does not stand for any type of bodily annihilation.

Privileging pollution

We saw in an earlier context (see Chapter 3) that in a cultural sense women drug users' bodies are represented as extremely polluted and bear the burden of being represented as less than moral, sexually loose and bad carers. And of course the notion of polluted body features strongly for women who use drugs during pregnancy. Here, while a drug-using women becomes the cultural representation of a woman who does not care about her body and is perceived as diseased, and an excluded citizen, her response can be that of disgust. Disgust, as Sara Ahmed (2004: 84) suggests, is an intense bodily feeling of being sickened, and disgust is always directed towards an object. For women drug users, the object can be plural and her disgust can be directed toward the person or persons (that is, partner, friend, treater, relative, and so on) who attempt to make her feel bad for being pregnant or, furthermore, wanting to be pregnant. The key thing about disgust is that the object must have got close enough to make us feel disgusted, and while disgust may take over the female drug user's body it will also take over the object (that is, partner, friend, treater, relative, and so on) (see Ahmed, 2004: 84).

The key question here is 'Why should a female drug user herself become the object of disgust when she can turn that disgust away from herself to those who unfairly judge her?' As Ahmed (2004) suggests, disgust brings the body close to an object only then to pull away from the object in the registering of proximity as an offence. So also the female drug-using body is able to pull away from partner, friend, treater, relative, and so on, and thus reject those who make her feel a bad, polluted body. In this way, she privileges pollution.

Embodying pleasure

We saw in Chapter 3 that, regardless of the perceived wisdom in the drugs field, pleasure is a part, if perhaps only a minute, if not small part of female drug use. Consistently in my work I have argued that it is important to look at the pleasurable effects of drugs side by side the tenderness which its painful consequences can evoke. In Chapter 3, I also outlined reasons why there has been a lack of interest in pleasure on the part of thinkers in the drugs field. But the main point I would like to emphasize here is that having pleasurable bodies is clearly experienced by female drug users. While this pleasure may be shaped by a conscious consumption in women's attempt to embody femininity, it is also a pleasure that is bounded by moralizing assumptions about the nature of drug use.

Perhaps in this context we can see that within the emotional economy of drug use, pleasure is distributed sparingly as a form of property, as a feeling drug users may have in the first place (see Ahmed, 2004: 162). For female drug users embodying pleasure means that they are aware that for most bodies in society pleasure is a must as a reward for good conduct, for bodies that are busy being productive and, in a heterosexual sense, reproductive. A woman drug user is viewed as neither productive nor reproductive, which is why she is not included in the pleasure economy. This is also why it is crucial for her to embody what little pleasure she can, not only from drugs but from her embodied life itself as a way of challenging her exclusion from full cultural pleasure. Of course, if poverty, violence, poor health and depression intersect with her embodied life, this task becomes very difficult.

The way forward

It has been my contention throughout this book that a feminist embodied approach would be useful to women drug users, clinicians and researchers alike. Consistently, I have suggested that we need to establish this new type of approach to replace outdated ideas but more importantly to maintain an anti-oppressive stance in which we complicate as well as theorize the concept of difference. Simply, when we treat difference as the basis for membership of society rather than as the site for social and cultural exclusion (Moosa-Mitha, 2005: 63), we cause trouble.

When we cause trouble in the drugs field, we learn to interrogate the normative assumptions and practices surrounding women's bodies that exist in both marginalized and privileged spaces. For example, we challenge the assumption that women's bodies are being contaminated and not worthy of reproducing. We reject the gender insensitive or racist practices which exist in many treatment agencies and which result in the unjust disciplining of racialized, gendered bodies. But we also ask why in the privileged space of theorizing in the drugs field, difference is rarely complicated. Rather it is taken for granted in a somewhat bland, individualistic way.

As we privilege difference, we privilege all those drug users, both women and men, who have the right to be equally unlike, different from or dissimilar to the embodied norms of White, male, Western bodies. Here the concept of difference is crucial. This concept is, as Rosi Braidotti (2002: 4) suggests, far too important to be left either to the geneticists or to the various brands of nostalgic supremacists (that is, White, male, Christian) who circulate these days. Given the 'conceptual acrobatics' (Reinarman, 2005) which exist in the drugs field, we need to make 'addiction specialists', both researchers and clinicians alike, feel uncomfortable if and when they reject a difference centred or feminist embodiment approach. While drug users can also be addiction specialists, it is of course in their interest to support this type of approach. Hopefully the discussions in this chapter and in previous chapters have helped the reader to generate an awareness of the usefulness as well as the need for a difference centred, feminist embodied approach and to see this approach as part of anti-oppressive theorizing.

In conclusion, *Revisioning women and drug use: gender, power and the body* has hopefully exposed the need for us to use the critical notions of gender, embodiment and power in the drugs field. In doing so, we bear witness to women drug users in order for them to maintain their corporeal integrity and self-worth. Let's help 'drug-using cyborgs' to emerge as a real political identity, embodied resistance and antagonist consciousness in the drugs field. Let's help all those refused stable race, gender or class membership to move away from the margins as they read 'webs of power'. Let's all cause some trouble and begin to change the world for women drug users with our conceptual armaments of gender, bodies, power, emotions and difference in hand.

Bibliography

Abercrombie P.D., and K.M. Booth (1997) 'Prevalence of human immunodeficiency virus infection and drug use in pregnant women: a critical review of the literature', *Journal of Women's Health*, 6, 2: 163–87.

Ahmed, S. (2004) *The cultural politics of emotions*. New York: Routledge.

Ahmed, S., and J. Stacey (2001) 'Testimonial cultures: an introduction', *Cultural Values*, 5, 1: 1–6.

Allen, B. (2006) 'Subaltern theories of health and illness: an ethnographic study of Mexican women with HIV disease', in V. Kalitzkus and P.L. Twohig (eds), *Bordering medicine*, Amsterdam: Rodopi, pp. 119–40.

Anderson, C., and D. Snow (1998) 'Reports of violence and relationship addiction: triggers to alcohol and other drug relapse', *Journal of Addictions Nursing*, 10, 1: 5–14.

Anderson, T. (1995) 'Toward a preliminary macro theory of drug addiction', *Deviant Behavior: An Interdisciplinary Journal*, 16: 353–72.

Anderson, T. (1998) 'A cultural identity theory of drug abuse', *Sociology of Crime, Law and Deviance*, 1: 233–62.

Anderson, T. (2005) 'Dimensions of women's power in the illicit drug economy', *Theoretical Criminology*, 9, 4: 371–400.

Anderson, T., and J.A. Levy (2003), 'Marginality among older injectors in today's illicit drug economy: assessing the impact of ageing', *Addiction*, 98: 761–70.

Anspach, R., and D. Beeson (2001) 'Emotions in medical and moral life', in B. Hoffmaster (ed.), *Bioethics in social context*, Philadelphia: Temple University Press, pp. 153–79.

Archibald, C.P., M. Ofner, S.A. Strathdee, D.M. Patrick, D. Sutherland, M.L. Rekart, M.T. Schechter and M.V. O'Shaughnessy (1998) 'Factors associated with frequent needle exchange program attendance in injection drug users in Vancouver, Canada', *Journal of Acquired Immune Deficiency Syndromes and Human Retrovirology*, 17, 2: 160–6.

Arfken, C.L., N. Borisova, C. Klein, S. di Menza and C.R. Schuster (2002) 'Women are less likely to be admitted to substance abuse treatment within 30 days of assessment', *Journal of Psychoactive Drugs*, 34, 1: 33–8.

Armstrong, D. (1987) 'Bodies of knowledge: Foucault and the problem of human anatomy', in G. Scambler, (ed.), *Medical sociology and sociological theory*, London: Tavistock.

Armstrong, D. (2002) *A new history of identity: a sociology of medical knowledge*, Basingstoke: Palgrave.

Baker, P. L. (2000) ' "I don't know": discoveries and identity transformation of women addicts in treatment', *Journal of Drug Issues*, 30, 4: 863–80.

Baker P.L., and A. Carson (1999) ' "I take care of my kids": mothering practices of substance-abusing women', *Gender and Society*, 13, 3: 347–63.

Balsamo, A. (1999) 'Public pregnancies and cultural narratives of surveillance', in A.E. Clarke and V.L. Olsen (eds), *Revisioning women, health and healing: feminist, cultural and technoscience perspectives,* New York and London: Routledge, pp. 231–53.

Barnett, T., and A. Whiteside (2002) *AIDS in the twenty-first century: disease and globalization,* Basingstoke: Palgrave Macmillan.

Bartky, S.L. (1990) *Femininity and domination,* New York: Routledge.

Barton, A. (2003) *Illicit drugs: use and control,* London: Routledge.

Bauman, Z. (1993) *Postmodern ethics,* Oxford: Blackwell.

Bean, P. (2004) 'Linking treatment services to the criminal justice system', in P. Bean, and T. Nemitz (eds), *Drug treatment: what works?* London: Routledge, pp. 219–35.

Bean, P., and T. Nemitz (2004) 'Introduction: drug treatment: what works?', in P. Bean, and T. Nemitz (eds), *Drug treatment: what works?* London: Routledge, pp. 1–18.

Belcher, J.R., J.A. Greene, C. McAlpine and K. Ball (2001) 'Considering pathways into homelessness: mothers, addictions and trauma', *Journal of Addictions Nursing,* 13, 3/4: 199–208.

Bell, N.K. (1992) 'If age becomes a standard for rationing health care . . . ' in H.B. Holmes and L.M. Purdy (eds), *Feminist perspectives in medical ethics,* Bloomington: Indiana University Press, pp. 83–90.

Ben-Yehuda, N. (1994) 'The sociology of moral panics: toward a new synthesis', in R. Coomber (ed.), *Drugs and drug use in society: a critical reader,* London: Greenwich University Press, pp. 201–20.

Bertin, J. (1995) 'Regulating reproduction', in J. Callahan (ed.), *Reproduction, ethics and the law,* Bloomington: Indiana University Press, pp. 380–97.

Berridge, V. (1998) 'AIDS and British drug policy: a post war situation?', in M. Bloor and F. Wood (eds), *Addictions and problem drug use: issues in behaviour, policy and practice,* London: Jessica Kingsley Publishers, pp. 85–106.

Best, S., and D. Kellner (1991) *Postmodern theory: critical interrogations,* New York: The Guilford Press.

Bloom, S.L. (2002) *The PVS disaster: poverty, violence and substance abuse in the lives of women and children,* Philadelphia: Women's Law Project.

Blum, L.M., and N.F. Stracuzzi (2004) 'Gender in the Prozac nation: popular discourse and productive femininity', *Gender and Society,* 18, 3: 269–86.

Bordo, S. (1990) 'Feminism, postmodernism and gender-scepticism', in L.J. Nicolson (ed.), *Feminism/postmodernism,* New York: Routledge, pp. 133–56.

Bordo, S. (1993a) *Unbearable weight: feminism, Western culture and the body,* Berkeley, University of California Press.

Bordo, S. (1993b) 'Feminism, Foucault and the politics of the body', in C. Ramazanoglu (ed.), *Up against Foucault: explorations of some tensions between Foucault and feminism,* London: Routledge, pp. 179–202.

Bourdieu, P. (1984) *Distinction: a social critique of the judgement of taste,* London: Routledge and Kegan Paul.

Bourgois, P. (1996) 'In search of masculinity: violence, respect and sexuality among Puerto Rican crack dealers in East Harlem', *British Journal of Criminology,* 36, 3: 412–27.

Boyd, S.C. (1999) *Mothers and illicit drugs*, Toronto: University of Toronto Press.

Boyd, S., and K. Faith (1999) 'Women, illegal drugs and prison: views from Canada', *The International Journal of Drug Policy*, 10, 3: 195–207.

Braidotti, R. (1994) *Nomadic subjects: embodiment and sexual difference in contemporary feminist theory*, New York: Columbia University Press.

Braidotti, R. (2002) *Metamorphoses: towards a materialist theory of becoming*, Cambridge: Polity Press.

Brain, O. (2006) 'Service user involvement: empowering users', *Druglink*, 21, 2: 6.

Bretteville-Jensen, A.L. (1999) 'Gender, heroin consumption and economic behaviour', *Health Economics*, 8, 5: 379–89.

Brook, B. (1999) *Feminist perspectives on the body*, London: Longman.

Brook, D.W., J.S. Brook, L. Richter, J.R. Masci, and J. Roberto (2000) 'Needle sharing: a longitudinal study of female drug users', *American Journal of Drug and Alcohol Abuse*, 26, 2: 263–81.

Broom, D. (ed.) (1994) *Double bind: women affected by alcohol and other drugs*, St. Leonards, Australia: Allen and Unwin.

Brown, L., and S. Strega (2005) 'Transgressive possibilities', in. L. Brown and S. Strega (eds), *Research as resistance: critical, indigenous and anti-oppressive approaches*, Toronto: Canadian Scholar's Press, pp. 1–18.

Brownmiller, S. (1984) *Femininity*, London: Paladin Grafton Books.

Brownstein, H.H. (1995) 'The media and the construction of random drug violence'. in J. Ferrell and C.R. Sanders (eds), *Cultural criminology*, Boston: Northeastern University Press, pp. 45–65.

Brunswick A.F., and P.A. Messeri (1999) 'Life stage, substance use and health decline in a community cohort of urban African Americans', *Journal of Addictive Diseases*, 18, 1: 53–71.

Bryson, V. (1999) *Feminist debates: issues of theory and political practice*, Basingstoke: Macmillan.

Buchanan, D., S. Shaw, W. Teng, P. Hiser, and M. Singer (2003) 'Neighborhood differences in patterns of syringe access, use and discard among injection drug users: implications for HIV outreach and prevention education', *Journal of Urban Health: Bulletin of the New York Academy of Science*, 80, 3: 438–54.

Buning, E.C., R.A. Coutinho, G.H. van Brussel, et al. (1986) 'Preventing AIDS in drug addicts in Amsterdam', *Lancet*, 1:1435.

Bunton, R., and R. Barrows (1995) 'Consumption and health in the "epidemiological" clinic of late modern medicine', in R. Bunton, S. Nettleton and R. Burrows (eds), *The sociology of health promotion*, London: Routledge, pp. 206–22.

Butler, J. (1990) *Gender trouble: feminism and the subversion of identity*, London: Routledge.

Butler, J. (1993) *Bodies that matter: on the discursive limits of 'sex'*, New York: Routledge.

Butler, J. (2004) *Undoing gender*, New York: Routledge.

Caan, W. (2002) 'The nature of heroin and cocaine dependence', in W. Caan and J. de Belleroche (eds), *Drink, drugs and dependence: from science to clinical practice*, London: Routledge, pp. 171–95.

Callaghan R.C., and J.A. Cunningham (2002) 'Gender differences in detox-ification: predictors of completion and re-admission', *Journal of Substance Abuse Treatment*, 23, 4: 399–407.

Callahan, J.C., and J.W. Knight (1992) 'Women, fetuses, medicine and the law', in H.B. Holmes and L.M. Purdy (eds), *Feminist perspectives in medical ethics*, Bloomington: Indiana University Press, pp. 224–39.

Campbell, N. (1999) 'Regulating "maternal instinct": governing mentalities of late twentieth century US illicit drug policy', *SIGNS: Journal of Women in Culture and Society*, 24, 4: 895–923.

Campbell, N. (2000) *Using women: gender, drug policy and social justice*, New York: Routledge.

Carter, C.S. (2002) 'Prenatal care for women who are addicted: implications for gender-sensitive practice', *Affilia: Journal of Women and Social Work*, 17, 3: 299–313.

Chacksfield, J. (2002) 'Rehabilitation: the long haul', in W. Caan and J. de Belleroche (eds), *Drink, drugs and dependence: from science to clinical practice*, London: Routledge, pp. 233–62.

Chambliss, D.F. (1996) *Beyond caring: hospitals, nurses and the social organisation of ethics*, Chicago: University of Chicago Press.

Chequer, P. (2006) 'Service user involvement: user involvement in Southwark', *Druglink*, 21, 2: 5.

Chermack, S.T., B.E. Fuller and F.C. Blow (2000) 'Predictors of expressed partner and non-partner violence among patients in substance abuse treat-ment', *Drug and Alcohol Dependence*, 58, 1/2: 43–54.

Chesler, P. (1994) *Patriarchy: notes of an expert witness*, Monroe, ME: Common Courage Press.

Chitwood, D.D., J. Sanchez, M. Comerford and C.B. McCoy (2001) 'Primary preventive health care among injection drug users, other sustained drug users, and non-users', *Substance Use & Misuse*, 36, 6/7: 807–24.

Clarke, A.E., and V.L. Olsen (1999) 'Revising, diffracting, acting', in A.E. Clarke and V.L. Olsen (eds), *Revisioning women, health and healing: feminist, cultural and technoscience perspectives*, New York: Routledge.

Cohen, S. (2001) *States of denial: knowing about atrocities and suffering*, Cambridge: Polity Press.

Collison, M. (1996) 'In search of the high life: drugs, crime, masculinities and consumption', *British Journal of Criminology*, 36, 3: 428–44.

Coomber, R., and N. South (2004a) 'Drugs, cultures and controls in compar-ative perspective', in R. Coomber and N. South (eds), *Drug use and cultural contexts 'beyond the West': tradition, change and post-colonialism*, London: Free Association Books, pp. 13–26.

Coomber, R., and N. South (eds) (2004b) *Drug use and cultural contexts 'beyond the West': tradition, change and post-colonialism*, London: Free Association Books.

Copeland, J. (1998) 'A qualitative study of self-managed change in substance dependence among women', *Contemporary Drug Problems*, 25, 2: 321–45.

'Council to dig up phone boxes – the new crack houses', *Druglink*, 2004, 19, 5: 2.

Coyle, S.L. (1998) 'Women's drug use and HIV risk: findings from NIDA's cooperative agreement from community-based outreach/intervention research program', *Women and Health*, 27, 1/2: 1–18.

Cross, J.C., B.D. Johnson, W.R. Davis and H.J. Liberty (2001) 'Supporting the habit: income generation activities of frequent crack users compared with frequent users of other hard drugs', *Drug and Alcohol Dependence*, 64, 2: 191–201.

Curet, L.B., and A.C. Hsi (2002) 'Drug abuse during pregnancy', *Clinical Obstetrics and Gynecology*, 45, 1: 73–88.

Cusick, L., A. Martin, and T. May (2003) *Vulnerability and involvement in drug use and sex work*. London: Home Office.

Dale, B., and P. Emerson (1995) 'The importance of being connected: implications for work with women addicted to drugs', in C. Burck and Bebe Speed (eds), *Gender, power and relationships*, London: Routledge, pp. 168–84.

Davis, D.R., and D.M. DiNitto (1996) 'Gender differences in social and psychological problems of substance abusers: a comparison to nonsubstance abusers', *Journal of Psychoactive Drugs*, 28, 2: 135–45.

Davis, K. (1997) 'Embody-ing theory: beyond modernist and postmodernist readings of the body', in K. Davis (ed.), *Embodied practices: feminist perspectives on the body*, London: Sage Publications, pp. 1–23.

Davis, R. (1997) 'Trauma and addiction experiences of African American women', *Western Journal of Nursing Research*, 19, 4: 442–65.

Davis, W.R., S. Deren, M. Beardsley, J. Wenston, and S. Tortu, (1997) 'Gender differences and other factors associated with HIV testing in a national sample of active drug injectors', *AIDS Education and Prevention*, 9, 4: 342–58.

Davoli, M. (1997) 'Establishing mortality rates from cohort data', in G. Stimsom, M. Hickman, A. Quirk, M. Frischer and C. Taylor (eds), *Estimating the prevalence of problem drug use in Europe*, Luxembourg, proceedings of conference jointly organized by Pompidou Group of the Council of Europe and the European Monitoring Centre for Drugs and Drug Addiction, pp. 137–44.

Dearling, A. (1999) 'Drugs, young people and the internet', in A. Marlow and G. Pearson (eds), *Young people, drugs and community safety*, Lyme Regis: Russell House Publishing, pp. 134–44.

de Belleroche, J. (2002) 'Molecular basis of addiction', in W. Caan and J. de Belleroche (eds), *Drink, drugs and dependence: from science to clinical practice*, London: Routledge, pp. 123–33.

De Gama, K. (1993) 'A brave new world? Rights, discourse and the politics of reproductive autonomy', *Journal of Law and Society*, 20: 114–30.

de la Hera, M., I. Ruiz Perez, I. Hernadez-Aguado, M.J. Avino, S. Perez-Hoyos, and J. Gonzalez (2001) 'Gender differences in HIV risk behavior of intravenous drug users who are not prostitutes', *Women and Health*, 34, 2: 1–13.

Denton, B., and P. O'Malley (1999) 'Gender, trust and business: women drug dealers in the illicit economy', *British Journal of Criminology*, 39, 4: 513–30.

Derks, J., M.A. Hoekstra, and C. Kaplan (1996) 'Netherlands', in M. Coletti (ed.), *Cost A6 (Evaluation of action against drug use in Europe)*, Rome: Cedis editrice, pp. 164–89.

Deville, K.A., and L.M. Kopelman (1998) 'Moral and social issues regarding pregnant women who use and abuse drugs', *Obstetrics and Gynecology Clini North America*, 25, 1: 237–54.

Di Nitto D.M., D.K. Webb and A. Rubin (2002) 'Gender differences in dually-diagnosed clients receiving chemical dependency treatment', *Journal of Psychoactive Drugs*, 34, 1: 105–17.

Ditton, J., and R. Hammersley (1996) *A very greedy drug: cocaine in context*, Amsterdam: Harwood Academic.

Douglas, M. (1966) *Purity and danger*, London: Routledge and Kegan Paul.

Douglas, M. (1987) 'A distinctive anthropological perspective', in M. Douglas (ed.), *Constructive drinking: perspectives on drink from anthropology*, Cambridge University Press, pp. 3–15.

Doyal, L. (2002) 'Gender equity in health: debates and dilemmas', in G. Bendelow, M. Carpenter, C. Vautier and S. Williams (eds), *Gender, health and healing*, London: Routledge, pp. 183–97.

Dunlap, E., B.D. Johnson, and L. Maher (1997) 'Female crack sellers in New York City: who they are and what they do', *Women and Criminal Justice*, 8, 4: 25–55.

Dunlap, E., S.C. Tourigny, and B.D. Johnson (2000) 'Dead tired and bone weary: grandmothers as caregivers in drug affected inner city neighborhoods', *Race and Society*, 3, 2: 143–63.

Durr, M. (2005) 'Sex, drugs and HIV: sister of laundromat', *Gender and Society*, 19, 6: 721–8.

Duster, T. (1970) *The legislation of morality: laws, drugs and moral judgment*, New York: Free Press.

Edwards, G. (1978) 'Drugs and the questions that can be asked of epidemiology', in J. Fishman (ed.), *The bases of addiction*, Berlin: Dahlem Konferenzen.

Edwards, G. (2004) *Matters of substance. Drugs: is legalisation the right answer or the wrong question?*, London: Allen Lane.

Edwards, G., M.A.H. Russell, D. Hawks, and M. MacCafferty (eds) (1976) *Drugs and drug dependence*, Farnborough: Saxon House/Lexington.

Ekanem, E.E., and A. Gbadegesin (2004) 'Voluntary counselling and testing (VCT) for human immunodeficiency virus: a study of acceptability by Nigerian women attending antenatal clinics', *African Journal of Reproductive Health*, 8, 2: 91–100.

Elwood, W.N., M.L. Williams, D.C. Bell and A.J. Richard (1997) 'Powerlessness and HIV prevention among people who trade set for drugs ("strawberries")', *AIDS Care*, 9, 3: 273–84.

Epele, M.E. (2002) 'Scars, harm and pain about being injected among drug using Latina women', *Journal of Ethnicity in Substance Abuse*, 1, 1: 47–69.

Erickson P.G., J. Butters, P. McGillicuddy, and A. Hallgren (2000) 'Crack and prostitution: gender, myths, and experiences', *Journal of Drug Issues*, 30, 4: 767–88.

Ernst, S., and L. Goodison (1997) *In our own hands: a book of self-help therapy*, London: The Women's Press.

Ettorre, E. (1989a) 'Women and substance use/abuse: towards a feminist perspective or how to make dust fly', *Women's Studies International Forum*, 12, 6: 593–602.

Ettorre, E. (1989b) 'Women, substance abuse and self help', in S. MacGregor, (ed.), *Drugs and British society*, London: Tavistock Press, pp. 101–15.

Ettorre, E. (1992) *Women and substance use*, Basingstoke: Macmillan.

Ettorre, E. (1994) 'What can she depend on: substance use and women's health', in S. Wilkinson and C. Kitzinger (eds), *Women and health: feminist perspectives*, London: Taylor and Francis, pp. 85–101.

Ettorre, E. (2002) *Reproductive genetics, gender and the body*, London: Routledge.

Ettorre, E. (2004) 'Revisioning women and drug use: gender sensitivity, gendered bodies and reducing harm', *International Journal of Drugs Policy*, 15, 5–6: 327–35.

Ettorre, E. (2005a) 'Gender, older female bodies and medical uncertainty: finding my feminist voice by telling my illness story', *Women's Studies International Forum*, 28: 535–46.

Ettorre, E. (ed.) (2005b) *Making lesbians visible in the substance use field*, New York: The Haworth Press.

Ettorre, E. (2006) 'Women, drugs and popular culture: is there a need for a feminist embodiment perspective?', in P. Manning (ed.), *Drugs and popular culture: drugs, identity, media and culture in the 21st century*, Cullompton, Devon: Willan Publishing.

Ettorre, E., and S. Miles (2001) 'Young people, drug use and the consumption of health', in S. Henderson and A. Petersen (eds), *Consumption of health*, London: Routledge, pp. 173–86.

Ettorre, E., and E. Riska (1995) *Gendered moods*, London, Routledge.

Ettorre, E., and E. Riska (2001) 'Long-term users of psychotropic drugs: embodying masculinized stress and feminized nerves', *Substance Use and Misuse*, 36, 9 & 10: 1187 and 211.

Evans, M. and E. Lee (eds) (2002) *Real bodies: a sociological introduction*, Basingstoke: Palgrave Macmillan.

Evans R.D., C.J. Forsyth, and D.K. Gauthier (2002) 'Gendered pathways into and experiences within crack cultures outside of the inner city'. *Deviant Behavior: An Interdisciplinary Journal*, 23, 6: 483–510.

Faden, R., N. Kass, and D. McGraw (1996) 'Women as vessels and vectors: lessons from the HIV epidemic', in S.M. Wolf (ed.), *Feminism and bioethics: beyond reproduction*, New York: Oxford University Press, pp. 252–81.

Fagan, J. (1994) 'Women and drugs revisited: female participation in the cocaine economy', *The Journal of Drug Issues*, 24, 2: 179–225.

Fagan, J. (1995) 'Women's careers in drug use and drug selling', *Current Perspectives on Aging and the Life Cycle*, 4, 2: 155–90.

Farnham, C. (1987) 'Introduction: the same or different?', in C. Farnham (ed.), *The impact of feminist research in the academy*, Bloomington: Indiana University Press, pp. 1–8.

Featherstone, M. (1982) 'The body in consumer culture', in M. Featherstone, M. Hepworth and Bryan Turner (eds), *The body: social process and cultural theory*, London: Sage Publications, pp. 170–96.

Featherstone, M. (1991) *Consumer culture and postmodernism,* London: Sage Publications.

Ferrell, J., and C.R. Sanders (1995) 'Culture, crime and criminology', in J. Ferrell and C.R. Sanders (eds), *Cultural criminology,* Boston: Northeastern University Press, pp. 3–21.

Finnegan, R. (1997) 'Storying the self: personal narratives and identity', in H. Mackay (ed.), *Consumption and everyday life,* London: Sage Publications in association with the Open University, pp. 65–111.

Fiorentine, R., J. Nakashima and M.D. Anglin (1999) 'Client engagement in drug treatment', *Journal of Substance Abuse Treatment,* 17, 3: 199–206.

Flax, J. (1990) *Thinking fragments, feminism, and postmodernism in the contemporary West,* University of California Press.

Flemen, K. (2004) 'Gimme shelter: Wintercomfort five years on', *Druglink,* 19, 5: 12–13.

Fortney, D. (1990) 'Drug use in pregnancy', *Minnesota Medicine,* 73, 4: 41–3.

Frank, A. (1991) *At the will of the body: reflections on illness,* Boston: Houghton Mifflin.

Frank, A. (1995) *The wounded storyteller: body, illness and ethics,* Chicago: University of Chicago Press.

Frank, A. (2004) *The renewal of generosity: illness, medicine, and how to live.* Chicago: University of Chicago Press.

Fraser, N., and L.J. Nicolson (1990) 'Social criticism without philosophy: an encounter between feminism and postmodernism', in L.J. Nicolson (ed.), *Feminism/postmodernism,* New York: Routledge, pp. 19–38.

Friedan, B. (1963) *The feminine mystique,* New York: Dell Publishing Company.

Friedman, J., and M. Alicea (2001) *Surviving heroin: interviews with women in methadone clinics,* Gainesville: University Press of Florida.

Gatens, M. (1992) 'Power, bodies and difference', in M. Barrett and A. Phillips (eds), *Destabilizing theory: contemporary feminist debates,* Cambridge: Polity Press, pp. 120–37.

Gearon, J.S., and A.S. Bellack (2000) 'Sex differences in illness presentation, course, and level of functioning in substance-abusing schizophrenia patients', *Schizophrenia Research,* 43, 1: 65–70.

Gilbert, M. (1970) 'Women in Medicine', in R. Morgan (ed.), *Sisterhood is powerful,* New York: Vintage Books, pp. 62–6.

Gilligan, C. (1987) 'Woman's place in a man's life cycle', in S. Harding (ed.), *Feminism and methodology,* Bloomington, Indiana: Indiana University Press and Milton Keynes: Open University Press (published jointly), pp. 57–73.

Goldstein, R.B., G.J. Mcavay, E.V. Nunes, and M.M. Weissman (2000) 'Maternal life history versus gestation-focused assessment of prenatal exposure to substances of abuse', *Journal of Substance Abuse,* 11, 4: 355–68.

Greberman, S.B., and D. Jasinski (2001) 'Comparison of drug treatment histories of single and multiple drug abusers in detox', *Addictive Behaviors,* 26, 2: 285–8.

Gray, M. (1998) *Drug crazy: how we got into this mess and how we can get out,* New York: Routledge.

Green, C.A., M.R. Polen, D.M. Dickinson, F.L. Lynch and M.D. Bennett (2002) 'Gender differences in predictors of initiation, retention, and completion in an HMO-based substance abuse treatment program', *Journal of Substance Abuse Treatment*, 23, 4: 285–95.

Green, A., S. Day, and H. Ward (2000) 'Crack cocaine and prostitution in London in the 1990s', *Sociology of Health and Illness*, 22, 1: 27–39.

Griffin, C. (1997) 'Troubled teens: managing disorders of transition and consumption', *Feminist Review*, 55: 4–21.

Griffiths, M. (2005) 'Workaholism is still a useful construct', *Addiction Research and Theory*, 13, 2: 97–100.

Hallam, E., J. Hockey, and G. Howarth (1999) *Beyond the body: death and social identity*, London: Routledge.

Haller, D.L., D.R. Miles and K.S. Dawson (2002) 'Psychopathology influences treatment retention among drug-dependent women', *Journal of Substance Abuse Treatment*, 23, 4: 431–36.

Hammer, S. (1975) 'Introduction', in S. Hammer (ed.), *Women, body and culture: essays on the sexuality of women in a changing society*, New York: Harper and Row Publishers, pp. 1–9.

Hammersley, M., J. Ditton, I. Smith, and E. Short (1999) 'Patterns of ecstasy use by drug users', *British Journal of Criminology*, 39, 4: 635–47.

Hammersley, M., F. Khan, and J. Ditton (2002) *Ecstasy and the rise of the chemical generation*, London: Routledge.

Hammersley, R., and M. Reid (2002) 'Why the pervasive Addiction Myth is still believed', *Addiction Research & Theory*, 10, 1: 7–30.

Haraway, D. (1991) *Simians, cyborgs, and women: the reinvention of nature*, New York: Routledge.

Harding, S. (1987a) 'Introduction: is there a feminist method?', in S. Harding (ed.), *Feminism and methodology*. Bloomington: Indiana, Indiana University Press and Milton Keynes: Open University Press (published jointly), pp. 1–14.

Harding, S. (1987b) 'Conclusions: epistemological questions', in S. Harding (ed.), *Feminism and methodology*, Bloomington: Indiana University Press and Milton Keynes: Open University Press (published jointly), pp. 181–90.

Hayes, P. (2004) 'Treating drug users: the role of the National Treatment Agency for Substance Misuse', in P. Bean, and T. Nemitz (eds), *Drug treatment: what works?* London: Routledge, pp. 211–18.

He, H., H.V. McCoy, S.J. Stevens and M.J. Stark (1999) 'Violence and HIV sexual risk behaviors among female sex partners of male drug users', *Women, drug use and HIV infection*, Binghamton: Haworth, pp. 161–75.

Henderson, S. (ed.) (1990) *Women, HIV, drugs: practical issues*, London: Institute for the Study of Drug Dependence.

Henderson, S. (1993) 'Fun, frisson and fashion', *International Journal of Drug Policy*, 4, 3.

Henderson, S. (1996) 'E Types and dance divas: gender research and community prevention', in T. Rhodes and R. Hartnoll (eds), *AIDS, drugs and prevention: perspectives on individual and community action*, London: Routledge, pp. 66–85.

Henderson, S. (1997) *Ecstacy: case unsolved*, London: Pandora.

Henderson, S. (1999) 'Drugs and culture: the question of gender', in N. South (ed.), *Drugs: cultures, controls and everyday life*, London: Sage Publications, pp. 36–48.

Hill Collins, P. (1999) 'Will the "real" mother please stand up?: the logic of eugenics and American national family planning', in A.E. Clarke and V.L. Olsen (eds), *Revisioning women, health and healing: feminist, cultural and technoscience perspectives*, New York and London: Routledge, pp. 266–82.

Hedrich, D. (2000) *Problem drug use by women: focus on community-based interventions*, Strasbourg: Pompidou Group's Cooperation Group to conduct drug abuse and illicit trafficking – drugs.

Hill, S.Y. (2000) 'Alcohol and drug abuse in women', in M. Streiner, K. Yonkers and E. Eriksson (eds), *Mood disorders in women*, London: Martin Dunitz, pp. 449–68.

Hinchliff, S. (2000) 'Mad for it: ecstatic women', *Druglink*, 15, 5: 14–17.

Hinchliff, S. (2001) 'The meaning of ecstasy use and clubbing to women in the late 1990s', *International Journal of Drug Policy*, 12, 5–6: 455–68.

Holland, J., C. Ramazanoglu, S. Scott, S. Sharpe, and R. Thompson (1992) 'Risk, power and the possibility of pleasure: young women and safer sex', *AIDS Care*, 4: 273–83.

hooks, bell (1996) *Killing rage: ending racism*, London: Penguin Books.

Howson, A. (2004) *The body in society: an introduction*. Cambridge: Polity Press.

Humm, M. (ed.) (1992) *Feminism: a reader*, New York: Harvester Wheatsheaf.

Humphries, D. (1999) *Crack moms*, Columbus: Ohio State University.

Hunt, G., and K. Evans (2003) 'Dancing and drugs: a cross-national perspective', *Contemporary Drug Problems*, 30: 779–814.

Hunt, G., K. Joe-Laidler, and K. Evans (2002) 'The meaning and gendered culture of getting high: gang girls and drug use issues', *Contemporary Drug Problems*, 29, 2: 375–411.

Hurston, Z.N. (1986) *Dust tracks on a road*, London: Virago.

Hutton, F. (2004) 'Up for it, mad for it? Women, drug use and participation in club scenes', *Health, Risk and Society*, 6, 3: 223–37.

Hutton, F. (2005) 'Risky business: gender, drug dealing and risk', *Addiction Research and Theory*, 23, 6: 545–54.

Inciardi, J.A., and L.D. Harrison (2000) 'Introduction: the concept of harm reduction', in J.A. Inciardi and L.D. Harrison (eds), *Harm reduction: national and international perspectives*, California: Sage, pp. viii–xix.

Irwin, K. (1995) 'Ideology, pregnancy and drugs: differences between crack-cocaine, heroin and methamphetamine users', *Contemporary Drug Problems*, 22: 613–37.

Jacobs, B.A., and J. Miller (1998) 'Crack dealing, gender, and arrest avoidance', *Social Problems*, 45, 4: 550–69.

Jainchill, N., J. Hawke and J. Yagelka (2000) 'Gender, psychopathology, and patterns of homelessness among clients in shelter-based TCs', *American Journal of Drug and Alcohol Abuse*, 26, 4: 553–67.

Jellinek, E.M. (1960) *The disease concept of alcoholism*, New Haven: Hill House Press.

Jewkes, R.J., and K. Wood (1999) 'Problematizing pollution: dirty wombs, ritual pollution and pathological processes', *Medical Anthropology*, 18, 2: 163–86.

Kalant, O.J. (1980) 'Introduction', in O.J. Kalant (ed.), *Alcohol and drug problems in women*, New York: Plenum Press. (Volume 5, *Research advances in alcohol and drug problems*), pp. 1–24.

Kaltiala-Heino, R., T. Lintonen, and A. Rimpelä (2004) 'Internet addiction? potentially problematic use of the Internet in a population of 12–18 year old adolescents', *Addiction Research and Theory*, 12, 1: 89–96.

Kandall, S.R., with the assistance of J. Petrillo (1996) *Substance and shadow: women and addiction in the United States*, Cambridge, Massachusetts: Harvard University Press.

Kaplan, T. (1982) 'Female consciousness and collective action: the case of Barcelona 1910–1918', in N. Keohane, M. Rosaldo and B. Gelpi (eds), *Feminist theory: critique of ideology*, Brighton, Sussex: The Harvester Press, pp. 55–76.

Kitzinger, J. (1994) 'Visible and invisible women in the AIDS discourses', in L. Doyal, J. Naidoo and T. Wilton (eds), *AIDS: Setting a feminist agenda*, London: Taylor and Francis.

Klassen, P. (2001) 'Sacred maternities and postbiomedical bodies: religion and nature in contemporary home birth', *SIGNS: Journal of Women in Culture and Society*, 26, 3: 775–810.

Klee, H., M. Jackson, and S. Lewis (2000) (eds) *Drug misuse and motherhood*, London: Routledge.

Knipe, E. (1995) *Culture, society and drugs: the social science approach to drug use*, Prospect Heights, Illinois: Waveland Press.

Kovach, M. (2005) 'Emerging from the margins: indigenous methodologies', in L. Brown and S. Strega (eds), *Research as resistance: critical, indigenous and anti-oppressive approaches*, Toronto: Canadian Scholar's Press, pp. 19–36.

Koester, S., K. Anderson, and L. Hoffer (1999) 'Active heroin injectors' perceptions and use of methadone maintenance treatment: cynical performance or self-prescribed risk reduction?', *Substance Use and Misuse*, 34, 14: 2135–53.

Langman, L. (2003) 'Culture, identity and hegemony: the body in the global age', *Current Sociology*, 52, 3/4: 223–47.

Lather, P. (1999) 'Naked methodology: researching the lives of women with HIV/AIDS', in A.E. Clarke and V.L. Olsen (eds), *Revisioning women, health and healing: feminist, cultural and technoscience perspectives*, New York and London: Routledge, pp. 136–54.

Lather, P., and C. Smithies (1997) *Troubling the angels: women living with HIV/AIDS*, Boulder: Westview/HarperCollins.

Laudet, A.B., S. Magura, H.S. Vogel and E.L. Knight (2002) 'Interest in and obstacles to pursuing work among unemployed dually diagnosed individuals', *Substance Use and Misuse*, 37, 2: 145–70.

Latka M., J. Ahern, R.S. Garfein, L. Ouellet, P. Kerndt, P. Morse, C.E. Farshy, D.C. DesJarlais and D. Vlahov (2001) 'Prevalence, incidence, and correlates of chlamydia and gonorrhea among young adult injection drug users', *Journal of Substance Abuse*, 13,1–2: 73–88.

Lee, E., and E. Jackson (2002) 'The pregnant body', in M. Evans and E. Lee (eds), *Real bodies: a sociological introduction,* Basingstoke: Palgrave Macmillan, pp. 115–32.

Lewis, S. (2002) 'Concepts of motherhood', in H. Klee, M. Jackson and S. Lewis (eds), *Drug misuse and motherhood,* London: Routledge, pp. 32–44.

Li, L., J.A. Ford, and D. Moore (2000) 'An exploratory study of violence, substance abuse, disability, and gender', *Social Behavior and Personality,* 28, 1: 61–71.

Littlewood, R. (2002) *Pathologies of the West,* London: Continuum.

Lombardi, E.L., and G. Van Servellen (2000) 'Building culturally sensitive substance use prevention and treatment programs for transgendered populations', *Journal of Substance Abuse Treatment,* 19, 3: 291–6.

Longhurst, R. (2001) 'Breaking corporeal boundaries: pregnant bodies in public places', in R. Holliday and J. Hassard (eds), *Contested bodies,* London: Routledge, pp. 81–94.

Lorber, J. (1994) *Paradoxes of gender,* New York: Yale University Press.

Lorber, J. (1997) *Gender and the social construction of illness,* London: Sage Publications.

Lorde, A. (1984) 'Age, race, class and sex: women defining difference', from *Sister outsider,* quoted in M.B. Zinn, P. Hondagneu-Sotelo and M.A. Messner (2005), *From gender through the prism of difference,* New York: Oxford University Press, pp. 245–50 (third edition).

Lupton, D. (1994) *Medicine as culture: illness, disease and the body in Western societies,* London: Sage.

Lupton, D. (1999) *Risk,* London: Routledge.

Lury, C. (1996) *Consumer culture,* New Brunswick, New Jersey: Rutgers University Press.

Lyon, M.L., and J.M. Barbalet (1994) 'Society's body: emotion and the "somatization" of social theory', in T.J. Csordas (ed.), *Embodiment and experience: the existential ground of culture and the self,* Cambridge: Cambridge University Press, pp. 48–66.

Macfarlane, A., M. Macfarlane, and P. Robson (1996) *The user: the truth about drugs, what they do, how they feel, and why people take them,* Oxford: Oxford University Press.

Mackay, H. (1997) 'Introduction', in H Mackay (ed.), *Consumption and everyday life,* London: Sage Publications in association with The Open University, pp. 1–12.

MacRae, R., and E. Aalto (2000) 'Gendered power dynamics and HIV risk in drug using sexual relationships', *AIDS CARE,* 12, 4: 505–51.

Maher, L. (1997) *Sexed work: gender, race and resistance in a Brooklyn drug market,* Oxford: Oxford University Press.

Mahowald, M.B. (1994) 'Reproductive genetics and gender justice', in K. Rothenberg and E.J. Thomson (eds), *Women and prenatal testing: facing the challenges of genetic testing,* Columbus, Ohio: Ohio State University Press, pp. 67–87.

Malloch, M.S. (2004) 'Not fragrant at all: criminal justice responses to "risky" women', *Critical Social Policy,* 24, 3: 385–405.

Markovic, N., R.B. Ness, D. Cefilli, J.A. Grisso, S. Stahmer, and L.M. Shaw (2000) 'Substance use measures among women in early pregnancy', *American Journal of Obstetrics and Gynecology*, 183, 3: 627–32.

Martin, B. (1992) 'Elements of a Derridean social theory', in A. Dallery, C.E. Scott and H. Roberts (eds), *Ethics and danger: essays on Heidegger and continental thought*, Albany: State University of New York Press, pp. 301–15.

Martin, E. (1992) *The woman in the body: a cultural analysis of reproduction*, Boston: Beacon Press.

Martin, E. (1994) *Flexible bodies: the role of immunity in American culture from the days of polio to the ages of AIDS*, Boston: Beacon Press.

Martin, S.E., and K. Bryant (2001) 'Gender differences in the association of alcohol intoxication and illicit drug abuse among persons arrested for violent and property offenses', *Journal of Substance Abuse*, 13, 4: 563–81.

May, T., M. Edmunds, and M. Hough, with the assistance of C. Harvey (1999) *Street business: the links between sex and drug markets*, London: Home Office.

Maynard, M. (1994) 'Method, practice and epistemology: the debate about feminism and research', in M. Maynard and J. Purvis (eds), *Researching women's lives from a feminist perspective*, London: Taylor and Francis.

Mazza, D., and L. Dennerstein (1996) 'Psychotropic drug use by women: could violence account for the gender difference?', *J Psychosom Obstet Gynecol*, 17, 4: 229–34.

McCoy, V., R. Correa, and E. Fritz (1996) 'HIV diffusion patterns and mobility: gender differences among drug users', *Population Research and Policy Review*, 15, 3: 249–64.

McCoy, C.B., J.M. Shultz, J.B. Page, E. Philippe, C. Mckay, and L.R. Metsch (1999) 'Gender comparisons of injection drug use practices in shooting galleries', *Population Research and Policy Review*, 18, 1–2: 101–17.

McDowell, L. (2003) *Redundant masculinities: employment change and white working class youth*, Oxford: Blackwell.

McKeganey, N. (2006) 'Street prostitution in Scotland: the views of working women', *Drugs, Education, Prevention and Policy*, 13, 2: 151–66.

McKeganey, N., and M. Barnard (1996) *Sex work on the streets: prostitutes and their clients*, Milton Keynes: Open University Press.

McKeganey, N., M. Barnard, A. Leyland, I. Coote, and E. Follett, (1992) 'Female prostitution and HIV infection in Glasgow', *British Medical Journal*, 305: 801–4.

McRobbie, A. (1995) *Feminism and youth culture*, Basingstoke: Palgrave Macmillan (second edition).

McRobbie, A. (2005) *The uses of cultural studies: a textbook*, London: Sage Publications.

McRobbie, A., and S.L. Thorton (1995) 'Rethinking "moral panic" for multi-mediated social worlds', *British Journal of Sociology*, 46, 4: 559–74.

Meehan, W., L.E. O'Connor, J.W. Berry, J. Weiss, A. Morrison, and A. Acampora (1996) 'Guilt, shame and depression in clients in recovery from addiction', *Journal of Psychoactive Drugs*, 28, 2: 125–34.

Measham, F. (2002) 'Doing gender – doing drugs. Conceptualizing the gendering of drug cultures', *Contemporary Drug Problems*, 29, 2: 335–73.

Measham, F., J. Aldridge, and H. Parker (2001). *Dancing on drugs: risk, health and hedonism in the British club scene,* London: Free Association Books.

Mertens J.R., and C.M. Weisner (2001) 'Predictors of substance abuse treatment retention among women and men in an HMO', *Alcoholism: Clinical and Experimental Research,* 24, 10: 1525–33.

Metsch, L.R., C.B. McCoy, J.M. Schulz, J. Bryan Page, E. Philippe and C. McKay (1999) 'Gender comparisons of injecting drug use practices in shooting gatheries', *Population Research and Policy Review,* 18: 101–17.

Miley, W.M. (2001) 'Use of abnormal and health psychology as topics in a classroom format to reduce alcohol and other drug abuse among college students at risk', *Psychological Reports,* 89, 3: 728–30.

Millar, G.M., and L. Stermac (2000) 'Substance abuse and childhood maltreatment – conceptualizing the recovery process', *Journal of Substance Abuse Treatment,* 19, 2: 175–82.

Miller, M., and A. Neaigus (2002) 'An economy of risk: resource acquisition strategies of inner city women who use drugs', *The International Journal of Drug Policy,* 13, 5: 409–18.

Miller, M., A. Eskild, I. Mella, H. Moi, and P. Magnus (2001) 'Gender differences in syringe exchange program use in Oslo, Norway', *Addiction,* 96, 11: 1639–51.

Monaghan, L. (2001) *Body building, drugs and risk,* London: Routledge.

Moosa-Mitha, M. (2005) 'Situating anti-oppressive theories within critical and difference-centered perspectives', in L. Brown and S. Strega (eds), *Research as resistance: critical, indigenous and anti-oppressive approaches,* Toronto: Canadian Scholar's Press, pp. 37–72.

Moran, L. (2001) 'The gaze of law: technologies, bodies and representation', in R. Holliday and J. Hassard (eds), *Contested bodies,* London: Routledge, pp. 107–16.

Morgan, P., and Joe, K.A. (1996) 'Citizens and outlaws: the private lives and public lifestyles of women in the illicit drug economy', *Journal of Drug Issues,* 26, 1: 125–42.

Mulia, N. (2000) 'Questioning sex: drug-using women and heterosexual relations', *Journal of Drug Issues,* 30, 4: 741–65.

Murji, K. (1999) 'White lines: culture, "race" and drugs', in N. South (ed.), *Drugs: cultures, controls and everyday life,* London: Sage Publications, pp. 49–65.

Mullings, J.L., J.W. Marquart, P.M. Diamond (2001) 'Cumulative continuity and injection drug use among women: a test of the downward spiral framework', *Deviant Behavior,* 22, 3: 211–38.

Murphy, S., and M. Rosenbaum (1999) *Pregnant women on drugs: combating stereotypes and stigma,* New Brunswick, New Jersey: Rutgers University Press.

Newcomb, M.D., and S.J. Rickards (1995) 'Parent drug-use problems and adult intimate relations: associations among community samples of young adult women and men', *J Couns Psychol,* 42, 2: 141–54.

Newman, K. (1996) *Fetal positions: individualism, science, visuality,* Stanford: Stanford University Press.

Nishimoto, R.H., and A.C. Roberts (2001) 'Coercion and drug treatment for postpartum women', *American Journal of Drug and Alcohol Abuse*, 27, 1: 161–81.

Oakley, A. (1997) 'A brief history of gender', in A. Oakley and J. Mitchell (eds), *Who's afraid of feminism?: seeing through the backlash*, London: Penguin Books, pp. 29–55.

Oaks, L. (2001) *Smoking and pregnancy: the politics of fetal protection*, New Brusnwick, New Jersey: Rutgers University Press.

O'Malley, P. and M. Valverde (2004) 'Pleasure, freedom and drugs: the uses of "Pleasure" in liberal governance of drug and alcohol consumption', *Sociology*, 38, 1: 25–42.

O'Neill, J. (2001) 'Horror autotoxicus: the dual economy of AIDS', in R. Holliday and J. Hassard (eds), *Contested bodies*, London: Routledge, pp. 179–85.

Orford, J. (2000) *Excessive appetites: a psychological view of addictions*, New York: John Wiley, second edition.

Paone, D., and J. Alpern (1998) 'Pregnancy policing: policy of harm', *International Journal of Drug Policy*, 9, 2: 101–8.

Parker, H. (2005) 'Normalization as a barometer: recreational drug use and the consumption of leisure by younger Britons', *Addiction Research and Theory*, 13, 3: 205–15.

Parker, H., F. Measham, and J. Aldridge (1995) *Drug futures: changing patterns of drug use amongst English youth*, London: Institute for the Study of Drug Dependence.

Parker, H., and F. Measham (1994) 'Pick 'n' mix: changing patterns of illicit drug use among 1990s adolescents', *Drugs: Education, Prevention and Policy*, 1, 1: 5–13.

Parker, H., L. Williams, and J. Aldridge (2002) 'The normalisation of "sensible" recreational drug use: further evidence from the Northwest England Longitudinal Study', *Sociology*, 36, 4: 941–64.

Parker, H., J. Aldridge, and F. Measham (1998) *Illegal leisure: the normalization of adolescent recreational drug use*, London: Routledge.

Patton, C. (1990) *Inventing AIDS*, New York: Routledge.

Patton, C. (1995) 'Between innocence and safety: epidemiologic and popular constructions of young people's need for safe sex', in J. Terry and J. Urla (eds), *Deviant bodies: critical perspectives on difference in science and popular cultures*, Bloomington, Indiana: Indiana University Press, pp. 338–57.

Pearce, J.J. (1999) 'Selling sex, doing drugs and keeping safe', in A. Marlow and G. Pearson (eds), *Young people, drugs and community safety*, Lyme Regis: Russell House Publishing, pp. 118–26.

Pearson, G. (1999a) 'Drugs at the end of the century', *British Journal of Criminology*, 39, 4: 477–87.

Pearson, G. (1999b) 'Drug policy dilemmas: partnership, social exclusion and targeting resources', in A. Marlow and G. Pearson (eds), *Young people, drugs and community safety*, Lyme Regis: Russell House Publishing, pp. 14–23.

Perry, L. (1979) *Women and drug use: an unfeminine dependency*, London: Institute for the Study of Drug Dependence.

Peters, T., and V. Preedy (2002) 'Alcohol and genetic predisposition', in W. Caan and J. de Belleroche (eds), *Drink, drugs and dependence: from science to clinical practice,* London: Routledge, pp. 27–37.

Plant, M. (1981) 'What aetiologies?', in G. Edwards and C. Busch (eds), *Drug problems in Britain: a review of ten years.* London: Academic Press.

Plant, M.L., M.A. Plant, and W. Mason (2002) 'Drinking, smoking and illicit drug use among British adults: gender differences explored', *Journal of Substance Use,* 7, 1: 24–33.

Plummer, K. (1988) 'Organizing AIDS', in P. Aggleton and H. Homans (eds), *Social aspects of AIDS,* London: The Falmer Press, pp. 20–51.

Plumridge, E.W., and S.J. Chetwynd (1999) 'Identity and the social construction of risk: injecting drug use', *Sociology of Health and Illness,* 21, 3: 329–43.

Probyn, E. (1990) 'Travels in the postmodern: making sense of the local', in L.J. Nicolson (ed.), *Feminism/postmodernism,* New York: Routledge, 176–89.

Purdy, L. (1996) *Reproducing persons: issues in feminist bioethics,* Ithaca and London: Cornell University Press.

Pursley-Crotteau, S., and P.N. Stern (1996) 'Creating a new life: dimensions of temperance in perinatal cocaine crack users', *Qualitative Health Research,* 6, 3: 350–67.

Raine, P. (2001) *Women's perspectives on drugs and alcohol: the vicious circle,* Aldershot: Ashgate.

Ramsay, M., and S. Partridge (1999) *Drug misuse declared in 1998: results from the British Crime Survey,* London: Home Office.

Reid, M., and M. Hammersley (2000) 'Sociopsychological issues in understanding gender relations and gender differences', *Psychology, Evolution and Gender,* 2, 2: 167–73.

Reinarman, C. (2005) 'Addiction as accomplishment: the discursive construction of disease', *Addiction Research and Theory,* 13, 4: 307–20.

Rhodes, T. (1997) 'Risk theory in epidemic times: sex, drugs and the social organisation of "risk behaviour"', *Sociology of Health and Illness,* 19, 2: 208–27.

Rhodes, T., and G. Stimson (1994) 'What is the relationship between drug taking and sexual risk? Social relations and social research', *Sociology of Health and Illness,* 16, 2: 209–28.

Rich, A. (1977) 'The theft of childbirth', in Claudia Dreifus (ed.), *Seizing our bodies: the politics of women's health,* New York: Vintage Books, pp. 146–63.

Rich, A. (1980) 'Toward a woman-centered university (1973–74)', in A. Rich, *On lies, secrets and silence: selected prose 1966–78,* London: Virago, pp. 125–55.

Richardson, D. (1993) 'AIDS and reproduction', in P. Aggleton, P. Davies and G. Hart (eds), *AIDS: Facing the second decade,* London: Falmer Press.

Richardson, D. (1996) 'Contradictions in discourse: gender, sexuality and HIV/AIDS', in J. Holland and L. Adkins (eds), *Sex, sensibility and the gendered body,* New York: St. Martin's Press, pp. 161–77.

Riess, T.H., C. Kim, and M. Downing (2001) 'Motives for HIV testing among drug users: an analysis of gender differences', *AIDS Education and Prevention,* 13, 6: 509–23.

Riska, E., and E. Ettorre (1999) 'Mental distress – gender aspects of symptoms and coping', *Acta Oncologica*, 38, 6: 757–61.

Roberts, A., M. Jackson, and I. Carlton-Laney (2000) 'Revisiting the need for feminism and Afrocentric theory when treating African-American female substance abusers', *Journal of Drug Issues*, 30, 4: 901–18.

Roberts, M., A. Klein, and M. Trace (2004) *Drug consumption rooms* (Drugscope briefing paper for the Beckley Foundation Drug Policy Programme, number 3), London: Drug Scope & The Beckley Foundation Drug Policy Programme.

Room, R. (1985) 'Dependence and society', *British Journal of Addiction*, 80: 133–9.

Rosenbaum, M., and K. Irwin (2000) 'Pregnancy, drugs, and harm reduction', in J.A. Inciardi and L.D. Harrison (eds), *Harm reduction: national and international perspectives*, California: Sage, pp. 89–109.

Rothman, B.K. (1989) *Recreating motherhood: ideology and technology in a patriarchial society*, New York: Norton.

Ruggerio, V. (1999) 'Drugs as a password and the law as a drug: discussing the legalisation of illicit substances', in N. South (ed.), *Drugs: cultures, controls and everyday life*, London: Sage Publications, pp. 123–37.

Rutherford, M.J., J.S. Cacciola, A.I. Alterman, and T.G. Cook, (1997) 'Social competence in opiate-addicted individuals: gender differences, relationship to psychiatric diagnoses, and treatment response', *Addictive Behaviors*, 22, 3: 419–25.

Sales, P., and S. Murphy (2000) 'Surviving violence: pregnancy and drug use', *Journal of Drug Issues*, 30, 4: 695–724.

Sbisa, M. (1996) 'The feminine subject and female body in discourse about childbirth', *European Journal of Women's Studies*, 3, 4: 363–76.

Scott, S., and D. Morgan (1993) 'Bodies in a social landscape', in S. Scott and D. Morgan (eds), *Body matters*, London: The Falmer Press, pp. 1–21.

Sedgwick, E. (1994) *Tendencies*, London: Routledge.

Seedhouse, D. (1998) *Ethics: the heart of health care*, New York: John Wiley & Sons, 2nd ed.

Segal, B. (2001) 'Responding to victimized Alaska Native women in treatment for substance use', *Substance Use and Misuse*, 36, 6: 845–65.

Shapiro, H. (2000) 'Wintercomfort: the price of trust', *Druglink*, 15, 2: 4–7.

Shapiro, H. (2005) 'Nothing about us, without us: user involvement past present and future', *Druglink*, 20, 3: 10–11.

Sheldon, S. (2002) 'The masculine body', in M. Evans and E. Lee (eds), *Real bodies: a sociological introduction*, Basingstoke: Palgrave Macmillan, pp. 14–28.

Sherman, S.G., C.A. Latkin, and A.C. Gielen (2001) 'Social factors related to syringe sharing among injecting partners: a focus on gender', *Substance Use and Misuse*, 36, 14: 2113–36.

Shidrick, M. (1997) *Leaky bodies and boundaries: feminism, postmodernism and (bio)ethics*, London: Routledge.

Shidrick, M. (2001) ' "You are there, like my skin": reconfiguring relational economics', in S. Ahmed and J. Stacey (eds), *Thinking through the skin*, London: Routledge, pp. 160–73.

Shilling, C. (1993) *The body and social theory*, London: Sage Publications.

Shilling, C. (2003) *The body and social theory*, London: Sage Publications (Second Edition).

Shilling, C. (2005) *The body in culture, technology and society*, London: Sage Publications.

Singer, M., G. Scott, S. Wilson, D. Easton, and M. Weeks (2001) 'War stories': AIDS prevention and the street narratives of drug users', *Qualitative Health Research*, 11, 5: 589–611.

Skeggs, B. (1997) *Formations of class and gender: becoming respectable*, London, Sage.

Sly, D.F., and K.S. Riehman (1999) 'Substance use, multiple substance use, sexual risk taking and condom use among low income women', *Population Research and Policy Review*, 18: 1–22.

Smart, C. (1984) 'Social policy and drug addiction', *British Journal of Addiction*, 79, 1: 31–9.

Smith, D. (1990) *The conceptual practices of power: a feminist sociology of knowledge*, Toronto: University of Toronto Press.

South, N. (ed.) (1999) *Drugs: cultures, controls and everyday life*, London: Sage Publications.

South, N., and D. Teeman (1999) 'Young people, drugs and community life: the messages from research', in A. Marlow and G. Pearson (eds), *Young people, drugs and community safety*, Lyme Regis: Russell House Publishing, pp. 69–80.

Spallone, P., and D.L. Steinberg (1987) 'Introduction', in P. Spallone and D.L. Steinberg (eds), *Made to order: the myth of reproductive and genetic engineering*, Oxford and New York: Pergamon Press.

Spittal, P.M., and M.T. Schechter (2001) 'Injection drug use and despair through the lens of gender', *Canadian Medical Association Journal*, 164, 6: 802–3.

Stabile, C.A. (1994) *Feminism and the technological fix*, Manchester: Manchester University Press.

Stanley, L. (1990) 'Feminist praxis and the academic mode of production', in L. Stanley (ed.), *Feminist praxis: research, theory and epistemology in feminist sociology*, London: Routledge, 3–19.

Stanley, L., and S. Wise (1990) 'Method, methodology and epistemology in feminist research processes', in Liz Stanley (ed.), *Feminist praxis: research, theory and epistemology in feminist sociology*, London: Routledge, pp. 20–60.

Stein, M.D., and M.G. Cyr (1997) 'Women and substance abuse', *Med Clin North Am*, 81, 4: 979–98.

Sterk, C. (1999) *Fast lives. Women who use crack cocaine*, Philadelphia: Temple University Press.

Sterk, C., K.P. Theall, and K.W. Elifson (2002) 'Health care utilization among drug-using and non-drug-using women', *Journal of Urban Health: Bulletin of the New York Academy of Medicine*, 79, 4: 586–99.

Stevens, S.J., and H.K. Wexler (eds) (1999) *Women and substance abuse: gender transparency*, Binghamton: Haworth Press.

Stevens, S.J., A.L. Estrada and B.D. Estrada (1999) 'HIV sex and drug risk behavior and behavior change in a national sample of injection drug and crack cocaine using women', *Women and Health*, 27, 1/2: 25–48.

Stevens, S.J., S. Tortu and S.L. Coyle (1998) 'Women drug users and HIV prevention: overview of findings and research needs', *Women and Health*, 27, 1/2: 19–23.

Stimson, G. (1990) 'AIDS and HIV: the challenge for British drug services', *British Journal of Addiction*, 85: 329–39.

Stocco, P., A. Calafat, and F. Mendes (2000) 'Preface', in P. Stocco, J.J. Llopis-llacer, L. DeFazio, A. Calafat and F. Mendes (eds), *Women's drug abuse in Europe: gender identity*, Palma de Mallorca: IREFREA.

Stormer, N. (2000) 'Prenatal space', *SIGNS: Journal of women in culture and society*, 26, 1: 109–44.

Strega, S. (2004) 'The view from poststructural margins: epistemology and methodology reconsidered', in L. Brown and S. Strega (eds), *Research as resistance: critical, indigenous and anti-oppressive approaches*, Toronto: Canadian Scholar's Press, pp. 199–235.

Tardiff, K., A.C. Leon, C.S. Hirsch, L. Portera, N. Hartwell, and P.M. Marzuk (1997) 'HIV infection among victims of accidental fatal drug overdoses in New York City', *Addiction*, 92, 8: 1017–22.

Taylor, A. (1993) *Women drug users: an ethnography of a female injecting community*, Oxford: Clarendon Press.

Teeman, D., N. South, and S. Henderson (1999) 'Multi-impact drugs prevention in the community', in A. Marlow and G. Pearson (eds), *Young people, drugs and community safety*, Lyme Regis: Russell House Publishing, pp. 99–108.

Terry, A., A. Szabo, and M. Griffiths (2004) 'The exercise addiction inventory: a new brief screening tool', *Addiction Research and Theory*, 12, 5: 489–99.

Thrift, N. (1997) ' "Us" and "them": re-imagining places, re-imagining identities', in H. Mackay (ed.), *Consumption and everyday life*, London: Sage Publications in association with The Open University, pp. 159–202.

Turner, B. (1986) *Medical power and social knowledge*, London: Sage Publications.

Turner, B. (1991) 'Recent developments in the theory of the body', in M. Featherstone, M. Hepworth and B. Turner (eds), *The body: social process and cultural theory*, London: Sage Publications, pp. 1–35.

Turner, B. (1992) *Regulating bodies: essays in medical sociology*, London: Routledge.

Turner, B. (1996) *The body and society*, London: Sage Publications, 2nd ed.

Tyler, I. (2001) 'Skin-tight: celebrity, pregnancy and subjectivity', in S. Ahmed and J. Stacey (eds), *Thinking through the skin*, London: Routledge, pp. 69–83.

Urla, J., and J. Terry (1995) 'Introduction: mapping embodied deviance', in J. Terry, and J. Urla (eds), *Deviant bodies: critical perspectives on difference in science and popular cultures*, Bloomington, Indiana: Indiana University Press, pp. 1–18.

Urla, J., and A.C. Swedlund (1995) 'The anthropometry of Barbie: unsettling ideals of the feminine body in popular culture', in J. Terry and J. Urla (eds), *Deviant bodies: critical perspectives on difference in science and popular cultures*, Bloomington, Indiana: Indiana University Press, pp. 277–313.

Vaarwerk, M.J.E.T., and E.A. Gaal (2001) 'Psychological distress and quality of life in drug-using and non-drug-using HIV-infected women', *European Journal of Public Health*, 11, 1: 109–15.

Valdez, A., C.D. Kaplan, and A. Cepeda (2000) 'The process of paradoxical autonomy and survival in the heroin careers of Mexican American women', *Contemporary Drug Problems*, 27, 1: 189–212.

Valliant, G.E. (1973) 'A twenty year follow-up of New York narcotic addicts', *Archives of General Psychiatry*, 29: 237–41.

Van Ameijden, E.J. (1992) 'The harm reduction approach and risk factors for human immunodeficiency virus (HIV) serocon-version in injection drug users in Amsterdam', *American Journal of Epidemiology*, 136: 236–42.

van Wormer, K., and D.R. Davis (2003) *Addiction treatment: a strengths perspective*, London: Thomson, Brooks/Cole.

Vogt, I. (1998) 'Gender and drug treatment systems', in H. Klingemann and G. Hunt (eds), *Drug treatment systems in an international perspective: drugs, demons and delinquents*, London: Sage Publications, pp. 281–97.

Waldorf, D., C. Reinarman, and S. Murphy (1991) *Cocaine changes: the experience of using and quitting*, Philadelphia: Temple University Press.

Walton, M.A., F.C. Blow, and B.M. Booth (2001) 'Diversity in relapse prevention needs: gender and race comparisons among substance abuse treatment patients', *American Journal of Drug and Alcohol Abuse*, 27, 2: 225–40.

Warburton, D.M. (1978) 'Internal pollution', *Journal of Biosocial Science*, 10: 309–19.

Watrey, S. (1987) *Policing desire: Pornography, AIDS and the media*, Minneapolis: University of Minnesota Press.

Wearing, B., S. Wearing, and K. Kelly (1994) 'Adolescent women, identity and smoking: leisure experience as resistance', *Sociology of Health and Illness*, 16, 5: 626–43.

Weeks, J. (1988) 'Love in a cold climate', in P. Aggleton and H. Homans (eds), *Social aspects of AIDS*, London: The Falmer Press, pp. 10–19.

Welle, D., G.P. Falkin, and N. Jainchill (1998) 'Current approaches to drug treatment for women offenders – Project WORTH', *Journal of Substance Abuse Treatment*, 15, 2: 151–63.

Wenzel, S.L., and J. Tucker (2005) 'Editorial: reemphasizing the context of women's risk for HIV/AIDS in the United States', *Women's Health Issues*, 15, 4: 154–6.

Westermeyer, J., and A.E. Boedicker (2000) 'Course, severity, and treatment of substance abuse among women versus men', *American Journal of Drug and Alcohol Abuse*, 26, 4: 523–35.

Wetherington, C.L., and A.B. Roman (eds) (1998) *Drug addiction research and the health of women: executive summary*, Roman A.B. Rockville, MD: National Institute of Drug Abuse.

White, E.F. (2001) *Dark continent of our bodies: Black feminism and the politics of respectability*, Philadelphia: Temple University Press.

Williams, S., and G. Bendelow (1996) 'Emotions, health and illness: the missing link in medical sociology', in V. James and J. Gabe (eds), *Health and the sociology of emotions*, Oxford: Blackwell Publishers, pp. 25–53.

Williams, S., and G. Bendelow (1998) 'In search of the "missing body": pain, suffering and the (post) modern condition', in G. Scambler and P. Higgs (eds), *Modernity, medicine and health: medical sociology towards 2000*, London: Routledge, pp. 125–46.

Williamson, J. (1989) 'Every virus tells a story: the meaning of HIV and AIDS', in E. Carter and S. Watney (eds), *Taking liberties: AIDS and cultural politics*, London: Serpent's Tail in association with ICA, pp. 69–80.

Willies, K., and C. Rushforth (2003) 'The female criminal: an overview of women's drug use and offending behaviour', *Trends and Issues in Crime and Criminal Justice*, No. 264 (October), Canberra, Australian Institute of Criminology. (webpage http://www.aic.gov.au/publications/tandi2/tandi264.html accessed 31 May 2005).

Wilson Cohn, C., S.M. Strauss, and G.P. Falkin (2002) 'The relationship between partner abuse and substance use among women mandated to drug treatment', *Journal of Family Violence*, 17, 1: 91–105.

Wincup, E. (2000) 'Surviving through substance use: the role of substances in the lives of women who appear before the courts', *Sociological Research Online*, 4, 4.

Wren, A. (2005) 'Keeping tabs on the herbal highs', *Druglink*, 20, 1: 16–17

Wright, S. (2002) 'Women's use of drugs: gender specific factors', in H. Klee, M. Jackson and S. Lewis (eds), *Drug misuse and motherhood*, London: Routledge, pp. 15–31.

Yanagisako, S.J., and J.F. Collier (2004) 'Toward a unified analysis of gender and kinship', in R. Parkin and L. Stone (eds), *Kinship and family: an anthropological reader*, Malden, MA: Blackwell Publishing, pp. 275–93.

Young, I.M. (1994) 'Punishment, treatment, empowerment: three approaches to policy for pregnant addicts', *Feminist Studies*, 20, 1: 33–57.

Index